The
Every
Other
Day
Diet

The Every Other Day Diet

The Diet That Lets You Eat
All You Want (Half the Time)
and Keep the Weight Off

KRISTA VARADY, PHD

AND

BILL GOTTLIEB, CHC

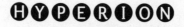

New York Boston

The advice herein is not intended to replace the services of trained health professionals, or be a substitute for medical advice. You are advised to consult with your health care professional with regard to matters relating to your health, and in particular regarding matters that may require diagnosis or medical attention.

Hyperion
Hachette Book Group
237 Park Avenue
New York, NY 10017

www.HachetteBookGroup.com

Printed in the United States of America

RRD-C

First Edition: December 2013
10 9 8 7 6 5 4 3 2 1

Hyperion is a division of Hachette Book Group, Inc.

The publisher is not responsible for websites (or their content) that are not owned by the publisher.

Library of Congress Control Number: 2013947671

ISBN 978-1-4013-2493-3

For my son, Gabriel; husband, Nicolas;
and parents, Eva and Lou.

—Krista

For my darling wife, Denise, who loves me every day.

—Bill

Contents

The
Every
Other
Day
Diet

Introduction

Welcome to the Every-Other-Day Diet

CUT BACK TODAY—
CUT LOOSE TOMORROW!

*D*iets *don't work.*

You've probably read that statement dozens of times, if not hundreds. But even though "Diets don't work" has become a truism, it's not true. The truth is *diets don't work when you diet every day.* Diets don't work because no one can endure day after day of deprivation, cut off from the foods they love. Diets don't work because no one can follow their complex and artificial rules for weeks and months on end. Diets don't work because they're unworkable!

But the reasons why traditional diets *don't* work are the

same reasons why the Every-Other-Day Diet *does* work—because it does away with daily deprivation and hard-to-follow rules. And you don't have to just take my word for it, because unlike other diets, the Every-Other-Day Diet has years of rigorous scientific research to back up its claims.

As a PhD in nutritional science and an associate professor of nutrition at the University of Illinois, I've spent the last 10 years conducting weight-loss studies on *modified alternate-day fasting*—a simple and science-proven approach to quick, permanent weight loss and lifelong weight maintenance. I've distilled that decade of systematic, successful research into a practical plan, which I'm presenting for the first time in this book, *The Every-Other-Day Diet*.

I want to take a moment to also introduce my coauthor, Bill Gottlieb, CHC, the author of 12 other health books that have sold more than two million copies worldwide, a health coach certified by the American Association of Drugless Practitioners, and the former editor in chief of Prevention Magazine Books and Rodale Books.

Bill not only brought his writing skills to *The Every-Other-Day Diet*; he also brought his skills as a veteran health journalist, working with me to find the latest scientific research, reported throughout the book. This book is infused with Bill's passion and professionalism as a health coach dedicated to the wellness of his clients and his readers.

In this introduction, I'll explain the difference between the Every-Other-Day Diet (the EOD Diet, for short) and the other diets out there. I'd also like to tell you my own story of losing weight by dieting every other day. Then I'll provide a brief overview of the contents of the book and how to use it for weight-loss success.

So let's get started with a closer look at the crucial differences between every-day dieting and the Every-Other-Day Diet.

FORGET ABOUT DIET DEPRIVATION—WELCOME TO DIET SATISFACTION

Every-day diets are typically about deprivation—what you *can't* eat. They tell you what *not* to do, handing down the dieter's equivalent of the Ten Commandments, like

- Thou shalt not eat more than 10% fat.
- Thou shalt not eat more than 40 grams of carbohydrates.
- Thou shalt not eat meat.
- That shalt not eat wheat.
- Thou shalt not eat sugar.
- Thou shalt not covet thy neighbor's sugar.

So you try to obey your diet's unique set of commands, whether there are 10 or 100 of them. But you end up feeling frustrated. So you "sin." You eat "bad" foods. You feel like a "bad" person. And then you repent. ("I'll never eat dough-nuts again!") And then, inevitably, you repeat the whole self-defeating cycle all over again.

Why does this happen? As day follows night, dietary excess always follows dietary deprivation. When a food is forbidden, it becomes tantalizingly tempting, and you crave it. Are you on a low-carb diet? You're probably craving pizza. On a low-fat, plant-based diet? You're probably dying for a steak. On a Paleo Diet? You're probably dreaming about cheese enchiladas. Eventually, you give in to those cravings. Maybe you even binge.

Another reason diets fail: hunger. Hunger is good. Hunger is *natural*. Hunger is your body's way of telling you that it needs fuel. The point of hunger is to let you know it's time to take in more calories. But weight-loss diets are about calorie restriction. (In spite of all the claims to the contrary by diet gurus who favor high or low quantities of carbs, protein, and/ or fat, it's *always* calorie restriction that powers a diet's ability to help you shed pounds.) So when you diet, you feel hungry. Maybe even cranky. Maybe even depressed. Nobody can deal with daily hunger and its accompanying emotional stress for long. The Every-Other-Day Diet solves this problem by making sure that you don't feel chronically deprived.

Diets also present you with a complex and daunting set of rules to be obeyed—or else. They tell you *what* you can and can't eat. They tell you *how much* you can and can't eat. They often tell you *when* you can and can't eat. All those rules end up ruling your life. And that's no fun. So what if you could drop pounds and still...

Eat all you want!

The Every-Other-Day Diet makes losing weight easy. There's no long-term deprivation, and there's one simple rule:

> **Eat 500 calories on the day you diet (Diet Day), and eat anything you want and as much as you want the next day (Feast Day).**

No keeping track of carbs, fat, or protein. No avoiding any particular food; all foods are allowed. No complex meal plans. And, yes, you diet only *every other day*. As I discuss at length in chapter 1, my research shows you lose just as much weight on the EOD Diet as when you're on an every-day diet.

With every-other-day dieting, dietary deprivation never lasts longer than a day, and total dietary freedom is always just a day away. Now, you may be thinking to yourself, "There's no way that's going to work. I'm going to eat so much on Feast Day that I'll never lose weight." But the studies I've conducted show that overeating on Feast Day *doesn't* happen. On average, people following the Every-Other-Day Diet eat about 110% of their normal caloric needs on Feast Day. And they eat about 25% of their normal caloric intake on Diet Day. That's an average of nearly one-third fewer calories over two days— and a perfect formula for steady, safe weight loss.

Why don't EOD dieters binge on Feast Day? Because they're not feeling deprived! When you're on the Every-Other-Day Diet, you know you'll be able to eat whatever food you want, and all the food you want, every other day. You don't have to eat "like there's no tomorrow" because there's a tomorrow right around the corner, and another one soon after that. The Every-Other-Day Diet solves the problem of diet *deprivation* with diet *satisfaction*.

MY PERSONAL STORY OF WEIGHT-LOSS SUCCESS ON THE EVERY-OTHER-DAY DIET

In this book you'll read many first-person stories from participants in my studies on the Every-Other-Day Diet, people who were officially classified as "obese" (about 30 pounds or more overweight) and who typically lost 20 or more pounds. But before I introduce you to those folks, I'd like to tell you my own story.

I've never had that much weight to lose, but, like most people, I sometimes struggle with extra weight. In the past, I tried to lose that weight with every-day calorie restriction. But the diet that I find works best for me is the same diet I've been studying for nearly a decade, the Every-Other-Day Diet. Here's what happened...

Back in 1996, at the age of 17, I was on my high school swimming team, working out for two hours at a time, up to 10 times every week. I needed a lot of calories to fuel those workouts (and my growing body), and I ate a lot. But I never had a weight problem. I was 5'7", 135 pounds, muscular, and strong. When I got to college, I stopped swimming competitively, but I kept on eating the same amount of food as I did in high school. It never occurred to me that the number of calories needed to power my workouts would be too many calories for my somewhat sedentary scholastic lifestyle. And so I gained about 15 pounds—the classic "Freshman 15."

Fortunately, I was majoring in nutrition, so I was learning for the first time about calories and healthier food choices. With that new knowledge, I started eating more sensibly, and slowly but surely I lost the weight I'd gained. By late in my sophomore year, I once again weighed 135 pounds. And that's right where my weight stayed until I was 31 years old and got pregnant.

The final trimester of my pregnancy coincided with the holidays. I found myself at party after party, feeling free to eat anything and everything I wanted to eat. (No one judges you for your appetite when you're pregnant!) As a result, I ended up gaining a little more weight than my obstetrician would have preferred, putting on about 40 pounds, rather than the suggested 25 to 35 pounds.

After my baby was born, I expected to easily lose that extra weight. And why not? Shedding extra pounds had been a breeze back in college. But I was in for an unpleasant surprise. About 25 of those extra pounds did come off quickly, which is pretty typical after a pregnancy. But the last 15? They stuck around. And I felt stuck.

Finally, after a couple of months, I put myself on a 1,300-calorie-a-day diet. And after six difficult months of daily deprivation, my weight was back down to 135. At that point, I figured the weight would stay off without my having to think about it. Wrong again. Over the next six months or so, the weight crept back on until I was back at 144 pounds. I couldn't believe it! I was eating healthfully. I was walking regularly. But here I was, overweight again.

Believe me, I didn't want to go back on a 1,300-calorie-a-day diet for months and months, endure the daily struggle, and hardly see the scale budge week after week. I was ready for a different approach. And so I started using the very same weight-loss method I'd been studying—the alternate-day modified fasting of the Every-Other-Day Diet. And like the participants in my studies, I loved it. I didn't have to diet every day. I could eat whatever I wanted to every other day, and I could eat as much as I wanted to. Best yet, I saw *immediate* results, quickly losing the weight I wanted to lose. I'm back to 135 pounds. And if I see the scale start to creep up by a couple of pounds—well, I just go on the Every-Other-Day Diet for a week or two, and the weight comes right off.

The Every-Other-Day Diet has worked for me. It has worked for hundreds of participants in my studies, all of whom have been 30 or more pounds overweight. And I'm sure it will work for you, a certainty I think you'll share after you read chapter 1 of this book, which presents the scientific evidence showing the effectiveness of the Every-Other-Day Diet. I feel quite passionate about my work and research, given the stakes: obesity is one of the biggest and most harmful health plagues of our time.

IT'S TIME FOR A REVOLUTIONARY APPROACH

The week I was finishing writing *The Every-Other-Day Diet*, the American Medical Association (AMA) decided to officially recognize obesity as a *disease*. (As a medical term, "obesity" is a reflection of body mass index, or BMI, a measurement of body fat. Medically, you're "overweight" with a BMI of 25 to 29.9, and "obese" with a BMI of 30 or over, which is generally 30 pounds or more overweight.) I certainly understand why the AMA made that decision.

Just about all of the participants in my scientific studies have been obese, so I know how difficult life can be for them. There's the discomfort of all those extra pounds. There's the struggle with self-esteem. And then there's the poor health: research links obesity to many other health problems, including heart disease, stroke, type 2 diabetes, cancer, osteoarthritis, gout, liver disease, sleep apnea, and depression.

In America, 36% of the population is obese and another 33% is overweight. Worldwide, 12% of the population is obese and another 22% is overweight. That's hundreds of millions of people worldwide who are weighed down by extra pounds. My sincere hope is that going on the Every-Other-Day Diet helps millions of them.

I began conducting research on modified alternate-day fasting because I knew that overweight and obesity were taking such a significant toll on the lives of so many people, and I saw that conventional, every-day diets were failing to help them.

I was looking for a new way, a better way, to first help people lose weight, and then to help them keep it off for a lifetime. My scientific research on both weight loss and weight maintenance shows that the every-other-day approach to weight control offers just the help overweight and obese people need. And I am delighted that now you'll be able to make practical use of my research by reading about and following the Every-Other-Day Diet and shedding those excess pounds once and for all.

How to Use This Book

Like the Every-Other-Day Diet itself, this book is simple to use. I suggest you do the following:

Start by reading chapter 1, which tells you about the scientific findings that support the EOD Diet. Chapter 1 will fill you with confidence and enthusiasm about this unique weight-loss program.

Next, read chapters 2 and 3 to orient yourself to Diet Day (500 calories) and Feast Day (unlimited calories). Once you've read them, you're ready to start the EOD Diet. But before you do, it will help to...

Check out chapters 4 and 5 for Diet Day ideas. Chapter 4 offers twenty-eight 400-calorie lunches, twenty-eight 400-calorie dinners, and twenty-eight 100-calorie snacks—all quick and easy to prepare, and all delicious. Chapter 5 guides you in selecting frozen, commercially prepared entrées that match the calorie requirements for Diet Day, and also offers snack ideas.

Read chapter 6 to turbocharge the EOD Diet with exercise. This chapter looks at my research on combining EOD dieting and exercise to help you lose more weight and lose it faster.

Keep the weight off with chapter 7. In this chapter, you'll find the Every-Other-Day Success Program, a science-proven way to keep off the weight you've lost. That's crucial, because five out of six dieters regain all their weight after one year. I'm happy to say that weight regain is unlikely to be your fate if you follow the EOD Success Program.

WELCOME TO FAST, EASY, AND PERMANENT WEIGHT LOSS

The Every-Other-Day Diet is simple and straightforward.

The Every-Other-Day Diet is easy.

The Every-Other-Day Diet is science-proven to *work*.

You'll lose weight fast and reach your goal weight.

You'll keep the weight off.

And you'll do so while eating all the food you want and any food you want, every other day.

Ready to get started? Just turn the page.

CHAPTER 1

The New Science of Every-Other-Day Dieting

Study after study shows the Every-Other-Day Diet really works

When it comes to health and wellness, there's a reason we look to the accuracy and authority of scientific experiments to help us suss out what's truly useful and sound information from all of the baseless, specious, and fad claims and advice out there—to separate the proverbial wheat from the chaff: *Scientific experiments aren't based on hype and hope.*

A well-designed, well-conducted scientific experiment helps separate truth from wishful thinking, fact from fantasy. And a *series* of scientific experiments, testing the same theory and generating the same results (what scientists call *replicating* a scientific finding), creates a body of knowledge you can *trust* and then *act on.*

Given the importance of weight loss to our health and well-being, to preventing and reversing disease, and to restoring self-esteem, you'd think most diet books would be packed with scientific evidence that justifies their approach. But that's *not* the way it is.

Yes, there have been scientific studies on a few popular diet plans. For example, a study published in the *Journal of the American Medical Association* showed that overweight and obese women on the Zone Diet, the low-carb Atkins Diet, or the low-fat Ornish Diet lost a little bit of weight after one year of dieting—an average of 3.5 pounds on the Zone Diet, 4.8 pounds on the Ornish diet, and 10.4 pounds on Atkins.[1] (Yes, that's after dieting for *one year.* I think you'll do a lot better on the Every-Other-Day Diet.) However, most popular weight-loss plans don't have any scientific support for their approach. None. Zero. Zilch.

Why am I making such a big fuss over scientific support for the diet plans in diet books? Because the Every-Other-Day Diet *does* have a significant body of scientific research behind it. To date, I've conducted seven clinical trials involving nearly 400 people, and I have published the results in 20 scientific papers. My studies have shown, again and again, that the Every-Other-Day Diet *works.* The people in my studies lose weight. And in my ongoing, three-year study on weight maintenance sponsored by the National Institutes of Health, EOD dieters are keeping the weight off.

In other words, the Every-Other-Day Diet is a research-proven diet that you can *trust.* If you follow this diet, eating

500 calories on Diet Day and whatever you want on Feast Day, the scientific evidence says you *will* lose weight. And if you go on the maintenance program described in chapter 7, the Every-Other-Day Success Program, my newest findings show you *will* keep the weight off.

I know the Every-Other-Day Diet may seem too good to be true. I know you might be asking yourself, "Can I really lose weight eating anything I want, every other day?" Never fear. You can. And not just because I say so—because nearly a decade of rigorous scientific research says so. And since your trust in the science-proven effectiveness of the Every-Other-Day Diet is so important to me, I've devoted this chapter to sharing the research and studies that support my claims. I want you to know—really *know*—that the diet you're about to undertake isn't a novel idea that's never been put to the test. It's not based only on the experience of patients in one doctor's practice (which is the case with many diet plans). And it's not theoretical—an idea that seems to make metabolic and biological sense, but has little real-world evidence to show that it works.

By learning about the science of every-other-day dieting and by reading about my studies and their positive findings, you can embark on this new weight-loss program with confidence, conviction, and enthusiasm. So let's start at the beginning: with my discovery of this diet, in the basement of a building on the campus of the University of California, Berkeley, where, in 2006, I was a postdoctoral fellow.

THE MICE THAT ALWAYS LOST WEIGHT

After I graduated from McGill University in Canada with my PhD in nutrition, I moved to California to do postdoctorate research in the Department of Nutritional Science at Berkeley. (A native Canadian, I was delighted to discover that "winter" in Northern California is just a series of rainstorms and that daffodils bloom in February!)

Under the guidance of my advisor, Dr. Marc Hellerstein, I investigated the effect of calorie restriction on cancer. There was already a lot of research on calorie restriction and longevity in animals; it showed that when mice are fed less food, they live up to twice as long as mice fed a normal diet. Furthermore, some of the biochemical mechanisms triggered by calorie restriction in longevity research are known to be anti-cancer. The mechanisms include slower cell division; lower levels of IGF-1 (insulin-like growth factor 1, a growth factor that stimulates cancer cells to divide and multiply); and lower levels of glucose, the main fuel for cancer cells.

Our research question was this: Can you put a mouse on the ultimate form of calorie restriction—fasting—so that the growth of cancer cells is slowed, but the animal does *not* lose weight? (In their research, scientists are always trying to isolate and analyze specific factors. In this case, we wanted to isolate the effect of *calorie restriction* on cancer from the effect of *weight loss* on cancer.)

But as hard as we tried, we couldn't keep the mice from losing weight! We fasted them one day and let them eat all they wanted the next day. But they never ate enough calories on "feed day" to fully compensate for the total lack of calories on "fast day." Sometimes they managed to eat 150% of a normal day's calories on feed day. Sometimes they ate up to 170%. But they never ate 200% of their normal caloric intake on feed day to make up for the zero calories on fast day. And so they *always* lost weight.

My experiment had failed because there was no way to separate the effect of calorie restriction from the effect of weight loss. I was not a happy scientist! But a scientific investigation that seems like a dead end can suddenly present a new vista of opportunity. And that's just what happened: I had a eureka moment, an *Aha!*, a conceptual breakthrough when I realized that the mice always lost weight on alternate-day fasting. The mice *always* lost weight. Could alternate-day fasting help us *humans* lose weight? If people fasted one day and then ate all they wanted the next day, would they always lose weight, just like the mice?

The concept of the Every-Other-Day Diet—using alternate-day fasting for *weight loss*—was born. It was time for me to say good-bye to the mice in the basement at Berkeley and move to Chicago, where I had been hired as an assistant professor in the Department of Kinesiology and Nutrition at the University of Illinois at Chicago. There, I started conducting studies on weight loss. With people.

THE MAGIC NUMBER

When I looked closely at the scientific literature on alternate-day fasting for cancer and heart disease—studies conducted exclusively on animals in the laboratory—I found that many of the risk factors for the two diseases were lowered most effectively when the animals ate only 25% of their normal calories on fast day. Not 75%. Not 50%. Not 0%, or a total fast. Time and again, the healthiest percentage was 25%, or what I call a *modified fast*.

And the 25% level of calories on fast day did more than prevent and reverse signs of disease. It also prevented the loss of muscle mass the animals otherwise had experienced at 0%, when they were given no food on fast day.

Why was that important? Losing muscle mass while dieting is a disaster for weight loss and weight maintenance. That's because muscle (*lean body mass*, in scientific terms) is metabolically active tissue that burns a lot of calories. Lose muscle during dieting and you'll burn fewer calories after dieting and regain your weight—as fat! This is perhaps the key reason why 5 out of 6 people who lose weight gain it all back (and then some). So I decided that on fast day— the day called *Diet Day* in the Every-Other-Day Diet—people would eat 25% of their normal caloric intake, or about 500 calories. I was ready to recruit participants and begin my study.

At this point, I have to make an embarrassing confession: even though I was about to conduct a study on every-other-day dieting in people, I didn't think the diet would work!

Why not? Well, many overweight people eat around 3,000 calories a day, and I couldn't imagine they'd be willing or able to eat only 500 calories every other day. And then there was my conversation at a medical conference with Dr. Eric Ravussin, PhD, director of the Nutrition and Obesity Research Center at the Pennington Biomedical Research Center at Louisiana State University. I told him I was thinking of conducting a study on alternate-day fasting for weight loss, allowing my participants to eat 500 calories on fast day.

"Don't even bother," he said. And then he proceeded to tell me (to my surprise) that he and his colleagues had recently conducted a human study on alternate-day fasting, in which the participants ate zero calories on fast day. A study that didn't go too well.[2] First, he wasn't able to recruit anyone from outside Pennington to participate in the study, because the idea of fasting every other day seemed so onerous; he was forced to enroll Pennington professors in the study. Next, he couldn't even convince many of those professors to participate for all three weeks of the study. Of the 16 that started, only 8 finished. And even those who finished told him they hated alternate-day fasting. Their families hated it, too. "I was so cranky and irritable on fast day that my wife wouldn't talk to me," said Dr. Ravussin, who participated in his own study.

I had already planned to allow my study participants to eat 500 calories on fast day; my conversation with Dr. Ravussin convinced me I'd made the right decision. For successful every-other-day dieting, you need to be on a *modified fast*, not a total fast. (In scientific papers, I sometimes call my approach ADMF, or alternate-day modified fasting.) You need to eat a small meal during the day, so you can stay balanced emotionally and mentally, interact with people without blowing a fuse, and get through your workday efficiently and effectively.

In spite of my doubts, I went ahead with my study, recruiting people who were normal weight and overweight (not obese). My goals for the study were broad: to find out if anyone could actually stay on the diet for a few months, and if they would lose weight. Much to my surprise, they did both!

There were 32 people in the original study.[3] Sixteen went on the Every-Other-Day Diet. The other 16 were the *control group*—they didn't diet or change their eating habits at all. After three months, my colleagues and I compared the two groups. Not surprisingly, people in the control group didn't lose any weight. But all of the every-other-day dieters shed pounds.

The folks who were normal weight at the start of the diet lost an average of 11.9 pounds after three months. Those who were overweight lost an average of 11 pounds. (A few of them lost as much as 25 pounds.) The overweight group also saw significant drops in bad cholesterol (low-density lipoprotein, or LDL) and in high blood pressure. And most of the participants said they didn't find the diet difficult at all.

I had proven to myself that every-other-day dieting was a reasonable, effective approach to weight loss. People *could* eat 500 calories every other day on Diet Days, without difficulty. People *could* eat whatever they wanted on Feast Day and still lose weight.

As you can imagine, I was very excited about this first set of results. After all, just about everybody hates daily dieting. Don't you? You hate the endless weeks and months of nonstop deprivation. You hate the constant hunger. You hate the complicated requirements and rules. That's why you've probably quit most of the diets you've started. Who wouldn't? Daily dieting is a drag. But every-other-day dieting is a new and effective way for people to lose weight—*without* deprivation, *without* hunger, *without* rigid rules.

After the success of this first study, there were many other questions about every-other-day dieting that I wanted to answer, with detailed, careful, and repeated research:

- Would the diet work on the obese, or would they binge on Feast Day?
- How hungry would obese people be on the diet? So hungry they couldn't help but overeat?
- Could people exercise on Diet Day? And would they overeat when they exercised?
- Would the diet work if you ate high-fat food? Or was low-fat food the only way to go?
- How would the diet affect risk factors for heart disease like total cholesterol, LDL cholesterol, HDL cholesterol, and high blood pressure?
- How would the diet affect hormones like leptin, which play such a key role in appetite?
- Was there a way for people who lost weight on the Every-Other-Day Diet to *maintain* their weight loss?

Nearly a decade later, after six more studies on people and more than 20 published scientific papers on every-other-day dieting, I'm proud and delighted to say that these questions have been answered. In fact, it's only *because* they were answered that I feel comfortable presenting the Every-Other-Day Diet to the tens of millions of people who *really* want to lose weight and keep it off and not just be disappointed by another every-day diet.

Let's take a closer look at a few of my studies and what I discovered. To make it easier for you to follow the trail of my research, I've listed the year each study was published, the journal it was published in, and the specific findings of the study.

BODY MASS INDEX—THE WAY SCIENTISTS MEASURE OVERWEIGHT

As you read the studies in the rest of the chapter, you'll encounter several common terms: *normal weight, overweight,* and *obesity.* However, nutritional scientists and other health experts use these terms in a very specific way: to indicate the level of *body mass index,* or BMI, a standard measurement of body fat. The three main categories of BMI are

Normal weight: BMI of 18.5 to 24.9
Overweight: BMI 25 to 25.9
Obese: BMI 30 and above

How do these three levels of BMI translate into actual pounds? Here are two examples: A 5'4" woman is normal at 130 pounds, overweight at 145 pounds, and obese at 174 pounds. A 5'10" man is normal at 160 pounds, overweight at 174 pounds, and obese at 209 pounds.

To figure out your BMI, use the BMI calculator at the website of the Centers for Disease Control and Prevention:

http://www.cdc.gov/healthyweight/assessing/bmi/adult _bmi/english_bmi_calculator/bmi_calculator.html

> Just enter your height in feet and inches, and your weight, and then hit the "Calculate" button. I'm happy to say my BMI is 21.6; my coauthor Bill's is 22.4. The Every-Other-Day Diet for weight loss, and the Every-Other-Day Success Program for weight maintenance, which you'll read about in chapter 7, helps both of us stay in the normal range.

2009, *American Journal of Clinical Nutrition*
The Every-Other-Day Diet works and is super-healthy, too!

A study in the *American Journal of Clinical Nutrition* was the first to definitively show that every-other-day dieting works to help obese people lose weight.[4]

My colleagues and I studied 16 obese people, 12 women and 4 men, with an average weight of 213.4 pounds and an average BMI of 33.8. All of them went on the diet for two months. For the first month, they ate frozen and other packaged foods for their 400- to 500-calorie lunches and 100-calorie snacks on Diet Day. (We distributed the lunches and snacks on a weekly basis.) For the second month, they prepared the Diet Day lunches and snacks themselves, after meeting with a nutritionist on our staff who counseled them about the calorie level of Diet Day and the foods and portion sizes that would help them stay at that level. (You'll find all the practical details for Diet Day in chapter 2.)

The results:

An average of 12 pounds of weight loss. After two months, the average weight loss was 12.3 pounds, a steady, healthy weight loss of 1.5 pounds per week. And the rate of weight loss was just about the same whether the participants were given frozen and packaged food or they prepared their own food. They just kept losing pounds, week after week.

Dieters lost fat, not muscle. Our EOD dieters also lost most of their weight as *fat*—11.9 pounds, on average, meaning that they shed only a few ounces of muscle. Losing fat rather than muscle is crucial in successful weight loss, because muscle burns calories. A typical dieter on other plans sheds 75% of her weight as fat and 25% as muscle; the typical EOD dieter sheds nearly all of her weight as fat. That's probably one reason why my subsequent studies have shown that EOD dieters, unlike most other dieters, don't regain the weight they lose.

Their BMI fell. The average BMI also dropped to 29.9. Many people who were classified as *obese* at the start of the study were now classified as *overweight*. That's a significant and health-giving improvement: as BMI decreases from obese to overweight, so does a person's risk for many diseases, including heart disease (obesity doubles risk), diabetes, arthritis, and cancer.

There was very little cheating. Our records showed that, on average, the dieters managed to meet the 500-calorie requirement of Diet Day for about 9 out of 10 Diet Days throughout the two months of the study. This showed me that the Every-Other-Day Diet is a diet people *could* and *would* follow at home.

Cholesterol plummeted. We also saw big decreases in total cholesterol (21 points) and LDL cholesterol (25 points), decreases that lower the risk for heart attack and stroke.

Dieters had lower blood pressure. Systolic blood pressure (the upper number of the blood pressure reading, reflecting arterial pressure when the heart pumps blood) dropped, on average from 124 to 116. Lower blood pressure means a lower risk for heart attack or stroke.

Dieters had a slower heart rate and a stronger heart. The participants also saw a startling drop in average heart rate, from 78 beats per minute to 74—a sure sign of a stronger, healthier heart.

My scientific conclusion: The Every-Other-Day Diet is an "effective diet strategy to help obese individuals lose weight and to confer protection against coronary artery disease." That's what I wrote (in the formal, restrained language of scientific discourse) in the *American Journal of Clinical Nutrition*.

For this book, I'll also state my conclusions about my studies a little more personally and enthusiastically: the Every-Other-Day Diet works—and it's really good for you, too!

PAUL'S STORY:
"I'VE GOT TO CHANGE MY LIFE."

Weight loss: 41 pounds

The evidence was conclusive for Paul Hussein, an international lawyer living in London and Switzerland. At 6 feet tall and 214 pounds, he was guilty of being overweight, and that extra fat—from eating a lot, and eating mostly high-fat food—was destroying Paul's health. His heartburn was so bad he had to take an antacid with every meal. He suffered from back pain. He had sleep apnea and snored. He felt tired all the time. He had type 2 diabetes and was on a medication to control his blood sugar. And he was a colon cancer survivor.

(continued)

In August 2012, Paul was watching the BBC documentary *Eat, Fast and Live Longer*, which featured my research on alternate-day modified fasting (the scientific term for every-other-day dieting) along with other methods of intermittent fasting. He told us what happened next.

"I said to myself, 'That's enough. I need to change my life—for myself, and for my wife and children. I need to go on a diet and lose weight.'"

Paul decided to go on the two-day-per-week pattern of dieting used by Michael Mosley, the program's host: a 500-calorie modified fast on any two days of the week, with unrestricted eating the other five days.

But the diet didn't work.

"I couldn't get a grip on my eating by fasting just two days a week," Paul told us. "I overate so much on the days I wasn't fasting that I didn't lose *any* weight."

So Paul went on the Every-Other-Day Diet. And this time, modified fasting worked. After nearly a year on the diet, Paul weighs 173 pounds—a loss of 41 pounds!

"One day of fasting followed by one day of feasting is the perfect diet for me," he said. And weight loss isn't the only positive change that Paul has experienced. His heartburn went away. He stopped snoring. His back pain is better. His blood sugar level has normalized, and he no longer needs to take diabetes medication. And at his most recent checkup for colon cancer, the doctor gave him a clean bill of health.

"I also find that I'm thinking a lot more clearly when I'm in court," he said. "And I don't feel tired during the day like I used to."

We asked Paul what he liked to eat on Diet Day. "I eat a simple vegetable soup, or perhaps a small piece of chicken with a serving of whole grain like quinoa and I feel very good after that meal. If I feel hungry on Diet Day, I drink a glass of water, or distract myself with another activity.

"Every-other-day dieting has now become my daily life and I don't think I will ever give it up."

2010, *Nutrition Journal*

Bingeing doesn't happen, hunger stops, and physical activity isn't a problem.[5]

Now I knew that every-other-day dieting *worked* for obese people. But I wanted to know more details about the diet:

- How hungry did people get on Diet Day, and was hunger a problem for trying to stick with the diet?
- Were people bingeing on Feast Day?
- Were people so physically depleted on Diet Day that they engaged in less physical activity?

To learn the answers to these questions, I analyzed some of the data from my first study more closely. I discovered the following:

There was no overeating on Feast Day. I thought the obese participants in my study would eat a lot more on Feast Day to make up for the caloric restriction of Diet Day, but they didn't. On average, the dieters ate the same number of calories they always ate (and even a little less), consuming an average of 95% of their normal caloric intake on Feast Day. In other words, Diet Day was *not* followed by Overdo-It Day!

Hunger vanished. My colleagues and I asked the study participants to rate their hunger on the evening of each Diet Day, using a scale of 0 to 100; 0 was "not at all" hungry, and 100 was "extremely" hungry. After three weeks of dieting, the average ranking was 60. After four weeks, it was 50. And after seven weeks it was 35. In fact, after about two weeks on the Every-Other-Day Diet, most of the participants said they felt little or even no hunger on Diet Day. That's more good news, because it's constant, gnawing hunger that drives most people to cheat on or quit a diet.

Satisfaction with the diet increased week by week. Meanwhile, over the eight weeks of the study, satisfaction with the Every-Other-Day Diet went up and up. Using the same 0 to 100 scale, the study participants reported a satisfaction level of 35 in the first weeks of the diet, but a satisfaction level of 50 by week eight. In other words, their good feelings about being on the diet—and no doubt their pride in the results as pounds kept peeling off—increased week by week. I'm pretty sure you'll have the same experience.

Physical activity wasn't a problem, even on Diet Day. We measured the level of physical activity throughout the study by asking the participants to wear a pedometer, a device that measures the number of steps taken every day. Two thousands steps is about one mile, and most of us take between 4,000 and 7,000 steps a day.

I thought the study participants would feel less energetic

on Diet Day and would take fewer steps. But that wasn't the case. The average number of steps on Diet Day and Feast Day were almost the same: 6,416 on Diet Day, and 6,569 on Feast Day. This was more good news: The Every-Other-Day Diet doesn't slow you down!

My scientific conclusions: "These preliminary data offer promise for the implementation of alternate-day fasting as a long-term weight-loss strategy in obese populations," I wrote in *Nutrition Journal*. I had made many additional discoveries about the Every-Other-Day Diet:

- Obese people could limit their food intake to one low-calorie meal and one snack per day and not overeat the next day.
- Hunger disappeared after two weeks or so on the diet.
- Physical activity didn't decrease on Diet Day.
- Weight loss was steady, constant, and significant.

My next and very important question: Could this diet help prevent and reverse heart disease? The answer, as you'll read in a moment, was an unqualified *yes*.

2010, Obesity

The Every-Other-Day Diet helps prevent and reverse cardiovascular disease—the #1 killer of people in the United States.

In my first study, the participants not only lost weight; they gained health.[6] Specifically, they gained added protection against heart disease:

A 21% decrease in total cholesterol. Their total cholesterol dropped from 175 to 138 mg/dL, for an average decrease of 21%. Every 1% drop in total cholesterol lowers the risk of heart disease by 2%, which means the Every-Other-Day Diet lowered the risk of heart disease by a whopping 42%. Not a bad "side effect" of successful dieting!

A 20-point drop in LDL cholesterol. LDL is the type of cholesterol that can build up on an artery wall and clog the artery, causing a heart attack or stroke. After eight weeks, the study participants had an average drop in LDL from 102 mg/dL to 72 mg/dL. This took them right to the 70 mg/dL level that doctors try to achieve in patients at risk for heart disease by prescribing a cholesterol-lowering statin like Lipitor or Zocor. (Personally, I'd rather lose weight than take a statin, since these commonly prescribed drugs are linked to fatigue, muscle pain, memory loss, and other health problems.)

Triglycerides fell from 125 mg/dL to 88 mg/dL. Like cholesterol, triglycerides are a blood fat that can raise your risk of heart disease. The study participants went from the "normal" to the "optimal" level of triglycerides, as defined by the US government's National Cholesterol Education Program.

Systolic blood pressure fell from 124 to 116 mm Hg. Eight points might not seem like much of a decrease, but it meant the difference between some of the study participants being prehypertensive—just below the level where a person would be diagnosed with outright high blood pressure—and having a normal blood pressure level, below 120.

My scientific conclusion: "Alternate-day modified fasting may decrease the risk of coronary heart disease in obese individuals," I wrote in *Obesity*, the world's leading scientific journal on the topic, in 2010. Given that heart disease kills 600,000 Americans every year, that's a very important finding.

THE EVERY-OTHER-DAY DIET IS SAFE

Over the years, I've often been asked about the *safety* of the Every-Other-Day Diet—after all, 500 doesn't seem like very many calories. Is it so few calories that EOD dieters could harm themselves in some way?

After studying hundreds of people on the EOD Diet, I'm happy to say that I've never seen a *single* health problem caused by the very low caloric intake of Diet Day or by the unlimited eating of Feast Day. Not a one.

In fact, I've seen just the opposite. Risk factors for heart disease normalize. Total and LDL cholesterol go down. Triglycerides decrease. Blood pressure is lower. Most importantly, of course, the pounds peel off—anywhere from 1 to 5 pounds per week, depending on how heavy the dieter was when he started the diet. And extra pounds are linked to a higher risk for dozens of different conditions and diseases, including cancer.

At the same time, unlike people on most other diets, the dieter doesn't lose calorie-burning muscle—and that retained muscle not only powers faster weight loss during the diet, but also sets the stage for postdiet weight maintenance. Many studies have linked increased lean body mass (muscle) to better health—even to longer life. So rather

(continued)

than posing a threat to health, the Every-Other-Day Diet improves health dramatically.

Of course, if you've got a chronic health condition like diagnosed heart disease, type 2 diabetes, or cancer, or if you're on any prescription medications, particularly drugs for controlling blood sugar, *you must check with your physician before starting the Every-Other-Day Diet or any weight-loss program.*

The EOD Diet (like most weight-loss diets) is not intended for pregnant women or women trying to get pregnant. It's also not for anyone with type 1 diabetes, where a modified fast might be harmful.

What about kids and teens? More than 30% of young people in the United States are now either overweight or obese. Could they benefit from the EOD Diet? The modified fast of the Every-Other-Day Diet isn't appropriate for the growing bodies of kids. However, I'm hoping to develop and study a version of the Every-Other-Day Diet for teens. Stay tuned, Mom and Dad!

Bottom line: The Every-Other-Day Diet is safe for just about everybody.

2012, Metabolism[7]

The Every-Other-Day Diet works even when you eat high-fat foods!

In my first two studies on every-other-day dieting, participants ate low-fat foods on Diet Day—because low-fat foods like fruits, vegetables, whole grains, and beans provide more filling bulk for fewer calories. But most Americans *don't* eat a low-fat diet. Just the opposite. They eat a high-fat diet, with 35% to 45% of calories from fat.

Since I wanted the Every-Other-Day Diet to work for everyone, I needed to find out if it could work for people who eat a high-fat diet on Diet Day while still maintaining the 500-calorie limit. To that end, I conducted a study with 32 obese people, putting them on the Every-Other-Day Diet for eight weeks. On Diet Day, 16 people ate high-fat foods that delivered 45% of calories from fat. The other 16 ate low-fat foods, with 25% of calories from fat. We prepared the foods for both groups, to guarantee their fat content.

The results:

The folks eating high-fat foods on Diet Day lost MORE weight than those eating a low-fat diet! That's right: after eight weeks on the diet, those eating high-fat foods had lost *more* weight than those eating low-fat food—9.5 pounds, compared to 8.2 pounds.

They had trimmer tummies. Both low- and high-fat groups trimmed nearly 3 inches off their waistlines. Dietary fat didn't make anybody fatter.

They had healthier hearts. Both groups had healthy decreases in total cholesterol, LDL cholesterol, and triglycerides.

My scientific conclusion: "An alternate-day fasting/high-fat diet is equally effective as an alternate-day fasting/low-fat diet in helping obese subjects lose weight and improve coronary heart disease risk factors," I wrote in the journal *Metabolism.*

Why did the people eating a high-fat diet lose more

weight? Well, they were slightly less likely to go off the diet on Diet Day, cheating 13% of the time, compared to 22% for the low-fat dieters. And I think it's likely they stuck to the diet *because* it was high-fat and therefore more enjoyable and satisfying.

Bottom line: The Every-Other-Day Diet works even if you eat high-fat foods on Diet Day. When it comes to weight loss, it's not fat that makes the difference. Or carbohydrates. Or protein. It's *calories.* Stick to the 500-calorie limit on Diet Day and you *will* lose weight.

2013, Obesity[8]

The combo of EOD dieting and exercise is unbeatable for weight loss and a healthy heart.

My first studies found that people didn't become less physically active when they were on the Every-Other-Day Diet, on either Diet Day or Feast Day. A modified fast didn't modify their capacity to move around. But, I wondered, what would be the effect of combining the Every-Other-Day Diet and *exercise*—not just daily physical activity, but a regular workout? Would people lose more weight than they would by dieting alone? Would their hearts be even healthier? My next study on the Every-Other-Day Diet attempted to answer those questions, by comparing people who went on the EOD Diet to people who went on the EOD Diet *and* exercised.

You can read all about this study in chapter 6, "Every-Other-Day Dieting and Exercise," but here's the super-positive bottom line: At the end of the study, folks who went on the EOD Diet and exercised had twice as much weight loss, had more muscle, banished more belly fat, lowered LDL cholesterol, and raised HDL cholesterol. The diet-alone group had only lowered LDL cholesterol.

My scientific conclusion: The combination of the Every-Other-Day Diet *and* exercise "produces superior changes in body weight, body composition [muscle and fat], and lipid [blood fat] indicators of heart disease risk, when compared to individual treatments," I wrote in *Obesity*.

Or, to put it less scientifically and more plainly: if you want the best results, go on the Every-Other-Day Diet *and* exercise.

2013 "ObesityWeek" (a presentation at the yearly scientific conference of the Obesity Society, which publishes the journal *Obesity*)

My NIH-sponsored research shows that the Every-Other-Day Success Program works—with this postdiet program, you don't regain the weight you just lost!

As I've pointed out several times in this chapter, the sad fact of weight loss is that it's almost never permanent. In a study published in the *International Journal of Obesity*, only 3% of people studied maintained their weight loss after five years. Other studies are a little more positive (but not much); they estimate that 80% to 90% of dieters regain all their weight.[9]

Unfortunately, most diet books ignore this fact. Or they make an enthusiastic but baseless pronouncement about how you'll maintain your weight after the diet. They might as well be telling you to believe in Santa Claus. I think any diet book that doesn't give you a science-proven, evidence-based program to *maintain* yourself at the weight you reached on the diet—and that's just about every diet book out there, including most of the other diet books on intermittent fasting—is setting you up for disappointment, not to mention the health problems that can go with regaining the weight you've lost. *The Every-Other-Day Diet* isn't that kind of diet book. It includes the Every-Other-Day Success Program, which you'll read about at length in chapter 7.

In November 2013, several months after completing the writing of this book, and six weeks before its publication, I reported the preliminary results of that study at the annual "ObesityWeek" conference, the world's most prestigious conference on obesity and weight loss.

Dieters had only 1 pound of regained weight. In the first six months of the study, people were on the Every-Other-Day Diet, and many people lost a lot of weight (up to 45 pounds). In the next six months, the folks who were on the EOD Diet went on the EOD Success Program. My preliminary results showed that they regained an average of *1 pound*. Meanwhile, the control group—people who went on a standard, every-day, calorie-restricted diet for six months and then went off the diet—regained an average of 5 pounds.

I'm also happy to say that all the heart-healthy benefits of the Every-Other-Day Diet—lower LDL cholesterol, lower triglycerides, and less belly fat—were maintained during the EOD Success Program. The participants also had lower levels of blood sugar and insulin, a sign that they were less prone to developing type 2 diabetes.

It's been a long journey from that basement at Berkeley

to a three-year, multimillion-dollar study sponsored by the National Institutes of Health; from the lightbulb of having a fresh idea to the light at the end of the tunnel for millions of people who have failed to lose weight on other diets, or who have shed pounds only to see their weight return.

My comprehensive research shows that the Every-Other-Day Diet is a wholly unique and effective way to lose weight and keep it off without daily deprivation, without hunger, and without complex and hard-to-follow rules. My research also shows the diet can help prevent and reverse several risk factors for cardiovascular disease, the #1 killer of Americans. And with all this positive research under my belt, I am very comfortable making you a promise about the weight you will lose on the EOD Diet.

WEEKLY, MONTHLY, AND TOTAL WEIGHT LOSS: THE EOD PROMISE

I'm sure you have one big question at this point: Just how much weight can I lose on the Every-Other-Day Diet? Well, I am happy to report that you can lose:

12 pounds per month. In my most recent research, many EOD dieters lost up to 12 pounds in the first four weeks of dieting, or 3 pounds per week—the promise on the cover of this book.

Up to 50 pounds. In my two- and six-month studies, some EOD dieters lost up to 50 pounds.

Of course, there's no *guarantee* you'll lose weight on the EOD Diet. In my studies, the rate of weight loss depended on how heavy my participants were when they started (the heavier you are, the more you lose); their level of motivation; and even the time of year when the study was conducted (it's harder to lose over the holidays). But if you eat 500 calories on Diet Day and whatever you want on Feast Day and stick to that pattern, it's nearly a certainty that you *will* lose weight at a steady rate, until you reach your weight-loss goal, whether that's losing 10, 25, 50, or 100 pounds or more.

And when you have reached your goal, it's time to implement the Every-Other-Day Success Program, the lifetime approach to keeping off the weight you just lost. You'll find the practical details of the Success Program in chapter 7. So what are you waiting for? Let's get started!

EOD—EASY AS 1-2-3!

1. The Every-Other-Day Diet has years of rigorous *scientific testing* behind it.
2. The Every-Other-Day Diet is *evidence-based*.
3. The results of the Every-Other-Day Diet are *real*.

CHAPTER 2

Diet Day

500 calories is easy, when it's every other day

Like other nutritional scientists, when I write up my studies for publication in journals, I almost never use the word *calorie*. Instead, I say *energy*, because that's what a calorie is: the amount of energy required to raise the temperature of one kilogram of water by one degree Celsius. Yes, a calorie is a measurable unit of heat, of energy, of *fuel*. If you ingest more calories than your body can burn, you store them (usually as fat)—and you gain weight. If you ingest fewer calories than your body needs to function, your body burns calories—and you lose weight.

Calories are the merciless mathematics of a food, of a meal—of a slim life, or a lifetime struggle with weight. And so we *count* calories, using books and apps and food labels and menus. And we *miscalculate* calories, gobbling up a low-fat food to shed pounds while overlooking the fact that it's sometimes loaded with high-calorie sweeteners. And we *debate* calories; a handful of experts claim that calories in some macronutrients like carbs burn differently than calories in others like protein or fat, spawning endless variations of low-carb/high-protein or high-carb/low-protein diets.

I think all those diets are high fad/low results. As a scientist who has devoted her professional life to studying calorie restriction, I can tell you with 100% certainty that if you eat food that contains less energy (calories) than your body requires, you will burn stored energy (calories) and lose weight. That's a scientific fact, like the law of gravity. Call it the Law of Calorie.

The Every-Other-Day Diet helps you obey the Law of Calorie in a completely new way. The Every-Other-Day Diet doesn't ask you to know and track the exact amount of calories in every food and beverage you ingest. (Good luck with that.) The Every-Other-Day Diet doesn't ask you to deprive yourself of calories every day, leaving you feeling hungry and frustrated. The Every-Other-Day Diet has one simple-to-follow, calorie-based rule:

Eat 500 calories one day (Diet Day)—and eat whatever level of calories you want the next day (Feast Day).

This chapter presents the practical details of Diet Day: how to successfully go through the day with minimum (or no) hunger and maximum chill. Want to start burning calories and losing weight? There's no time like Diet Day.

How Low Can You Go?

When you're not on a diet—when your every-day pattern of eating is aimed at *maintaining* weight—you probably consume somewhere between 2,000 and 2,500 calories a day. (The US government's Recommended Daily Allowance [RDA] for calories is 1,600 to 2,400 calories for women, depending on age and activity; and 2,000 to 3,000 for men.)

When you go on a diet—when you want to burn more calories than you consume and shed pounds—you submit to the eating pattern nutritional scientists call *calorie restriction*, usually limiting your daily intake to 1,000 to 1,500 calories a day. Some dieters, however, decide to consume even *fewer* calories. Why?

Maybe they're extremely obese, with 100 or more pounds to lose. Maybe they want to lose weight very quickly. And so they go on a *very low-calorie diet* (VLCD), with a daily intake of about 800 calories.

And then there's the Every-Other-Day Diet, where, on Diet Day, you consume 500 calories. Is that doable? Is that even *safe*? Yes and yes. Surprisingly, 500 calories can provide a lot of hearty eating: one (or even two) satisfying meals a day, along with a snack. Find that statement hard to believe? Just check out the yummy recipes and meal suggestions in chapters 4 and 5. You'll soon find that Diet Day is very doable and very delicious.

Some folks feel hungry on Diet Day for the first week or

two of EOD dieting. (Later in this chapter you'll find plenty of tips to help you get through the hunger pangs of those first few weeks.) But my studies show that the hunger quickly resolves: the folks in my studies report they *don't* feel hungry on Diet Day after two weeks or so on the diet. Hunger just goes away.

Bottom line: The experiences of hundreds of EOD dieters show that one day of modified fasting isn't all that hard— particularly when it's followed by a day of all-out dietary delight.

WHY 500 CALORIES?

As I discussed in chapter 1, my first scientific studies on alternate-day fasting for weight loss—the genesis of the Every-Other-Day Diet—were on mice. These studies tested many different levels of alternate-day calorie restriction, trying to determine the perfect level for healthy weight loss. I tried 75% of normal caloric intake; 50%; even 0%—a total fast. And the winner was 25%.

At 25%, the mice had the *maximal* amount of weight loss with the *minimal* level of muscle loss. In other words, they lost fat but not muscle. And retaining muscle while dieting is a must for health and long-term weight maintenance. Also, 25% of calories also produced the best improvements in risk factors for heart disease and type 2 diabetes.

Subsequently, my studies on people have confirmed that 25% is the perfect percentage for every-other-day dieting: 500 calories, if you normally eat 2,000 calories a day. At that percentage, you lose weight quickly, steadily, and healthfully.

Obviously, 25% of normal caloric intake is a different number for different people. If you're a 6'3" man weighing 205 pounds, the normal level of calories you burn is a lot different than if you're a 5'2" woman weighing 150 pounds; the bigger the person, the more calories needed to maintain weight. In my scientific studies with groups of people, we carefully determine 25% of normal caloric intake for each study participant, using a precise formula and double-checking it with a sophisticated medical test.

Unfortunately, I can't offer you that kind of individualized determination of 25% of your normal caloric intake; it's just not possible outside of a highly controlled scientific experiment. But here's the good news: an individualized version of the EOD Diet is *not* required for it to work. Why not? Because my studies have allowed me to determine a consistent average caloric intake on Diet Day: 480 calories for women and 520 calories for men. You don't need a degree in mathematics to figure out the average of those two numbers is 500. Which means that

- 500 calories on Diet Day is the average amount of intake among the hundreds of people who have participated in my studies and successfully lost weight;
- 500 calories is the *science-proven* level of calories for efficient weight loss; and
- 500 calories is the level that *works*, no matter what you weigh when you start the Every-Other-Day Diet. And you should weigh yourself when you start the diet and every day thereafter.

EIGHT TIPS TO MAKE DIET DAY WORK FOR YOU

Tip 1: Weigh Yourself Every Day

How often should you check your weight when you're on the Every-Other-Day Diet? In my studies, we encouraged the participants to weigh themselves *every day*, and to average the weight of the most recent Diet Day and Feast Day. For example, if you weigh yourself the morning of Diet Day and you weigh 148 pounds and you weigh yourself the morning of Feast Day and you weigh 150 pounds, your current weight is 149 pounds.

Why do I think you should weigh yourself every day? Maybe you've heard that you *shouldn't* get on the scale every morning, because it can be discouraging to discover you haven't lost much weight, or that it keeps your focus on short-term success rather than on permanent weight loss. But that's not what scientific studies show. They are *pro*-scale. Here are some very revealing results:

After one month of weighing, participants had 3 extra pounds of weight loss.[1] When researchers at the Minneapolis Heart Institute studied 100 obese people over six months, they found that people lost *1 pound more* for every 11 days they self-weighed. In other words, if you weigh yourself every day for a month, you lose about 3 pounds more than folks who don't. In fact, the folks who self-weighed were *10 times more likely* to lose at least 5% of their body weight during the six months of the study. "Self-weighing may be a strategy to enhance...weight-loss programs," wrote the researchers in the *American Journal of Preventive Medicine*. I agree!

When those same researchers reviewed 12 studies on self-weighing and weight loss, they found that 11 of the studies showed that self-weighing was linked to more weight loss and better weight maintenance, and also to not becoming overweight in the first place.

Daily weighing doubles weight loss. In a two-year study of more than 1,200 obese people conducted by scientists at the Marshfield Clinic Research Foundation in Wisconsin and reported in the *International Journal of Behavioral Medicine*, those who weighed themselves daily lost more than twice as much weight as those who weighed themselves monthly.[2]

People average 347 fewer calories per day when they weigh themselves that day. A team of scientists from the University of North Carolina studied 91 overweight people for six months, in an experiment focused on self-weighing.[3] Those who weighed themselves daily ate an average of 347 fewer calories per day than those who weighed themselves weekly. They also lost a lot more weight—17 pounds compared to four-fifths of a pound! The researchers also noted that the study participants who weighed themselves just about every day *liked* doing so. I think you will, too, as your scale gives you the most important and positive feedback of all: You are steadily losing the weight you want to lose! But weighing yourself daily is important not only for *losing* weight. It's also important for *maintaining* weight loss.

If people didn't weigh themselves regularly, 4.5 times more weight was regained. Researchers in the Department of Psychology at Drexel University conducted a one-year study on 3,000 people who had lost 30 pounds and kept it off for one year and reported their findings in *Obesity* in 2007.[4] At the start of the study, 36% said they weighed themselves at least once a day, and those who did so had the lowest body mass index (BMI, a standard measurement of body fat). They also scored highest on psychological tests measuring the ability to make rational choices about eating.

A year later, the researchers found that the change in the rate of self-weighing after the start of the study—whether or not the participants weighed themselves with lesser or greater frequency during the year of the study—was an *exact match* for the amount of weight regained:

- Those who self-weighed *less* regained 9 pounds.
- Those who self-weighed *at the same rate* regained 4 pounds.
- Those who self-weighed *more* regained 2 pounds.

"Consistent self-weighing may help individuals maintain their successful weight loss by allowing them to catch weight gains before they escalate, and make behavior changes to prevent additional weight gain," concluded the researchers in *Obesity*.

That's certainly my experience and my coauthor Bill's also. When I was cutting back on calories to lose weight after my pregnancy, I found that self-weighing helped me cheat less. I'd think, "Yes, I want that extra scoop of ice cream, but I have to face the scale tomorrow!" Bill is also a big fan of daily self-weighing, saying it's a big reason why he still weighs what he weighed in college. When the numbers on his scale start to go up, he makes sure his calorie intake goes down. In his role as a health coach, he counsels his clients to do the same.

Daily weighing is valuable. In another study, researchers at the University of Minnesota tracked more than 3,000 people over two years—some in a weight-loss program and some in a weight-maintenance program. Those who self-weighed the most during those two years had the *largest weight loss* in the weight-loss program, and the *smallest weight gain* in the maintenance program.[5]

"Daily weighing is valuable to individuals trying to lose weight or prevent weight gain," wrote the researchers in the *Annals of Behavioral Medicine.* "Daily self-weighing should be emphasized in clinical and public health messages about weight control." (That's why I'm emphasizing it here!)

When should you weigh yourself? Do it at the same time every day, because weight varies during the day. First thing in the morning—before you've had anything to eat or drink—is ideal.

FRED'S STORY: "THIS DIET HAS BEEN PERFECT FOR ME."

Weight loss: 30 pounds

"The Every-Other-Day Diet has been perfect for me," said Fred Lang, a marketing consultant in Chicago. "When I'm not on a diet, I normally skip breakfast, and eat a late lunch and a late dinner. So when I heard about Diet Day and Feast Day, the pattern of eating seemed a perfect match with my lifestyle. And it was. I found it very easy to have one

(continued)

meal on Diet Day, and then to just relax and eat anything I wanted to on Feast Day. On Diet Day, I made sure to drink plenty of water, which helped with hunger. I also drank diet soda, chewed gum, and had the occasional cup of coffee— all of which have zero calories. I ate one meal—usually a Lean Cuisine entrée, which was pretty good—and I had a nice snack later in the day. Plus, I knew that however hungry I felt, I would be eating plenty tomorrow.

"Mind you, I didn't have a ton of weight to lose—I'm 5'10" and weighed 190 pounds. But after 12 weeks of EOD dieting I'd lost *all* my extra weight—I'd shed 30 pounds and weighed 160. I can tell you, both me *and* my wife are really happy about that!"

Tip 2: Eat Lunch or Dinner (but Not Breakfast)

All the participants in my studies on the Every-Other-Day Diet have eaten *lunch* as their Diet Day meal. It's not that I think eating at noon is somehow crucial to losing weight. Rather, using the same Diet Day meal from study to study has allowed me to compare the results of all my various studies, instead of introducing another scientific variable (mealtime) that would make those comparisons more problematic.

If you want to match the methodology of my studies—if you want the highest level of confidence that the pattern of eating you're using is the same pattern scientifically shown to produce steady, significant weight loss—then eat *lunch* on Diet Day.

However, it's quite likely that the success of EOD dieting isn't tied to eating lunch. It's tied to a modified fast on

Diet Day and unlimited eating on Feast Day. So if you prefer to eat *dinner* on Diet Day—enjoying dinnertime with your spouse, family, or friends—go right ahead. But I do strongly advise against eating *breakfast* as your main meal on Diet Day, because you may find yourself so hungry by dinnertime that you won't be able to limit yourself to 500 calories for the day. I'm currently conducting a study using lunch *or* dinner as the meal on Diet Day, to see if people eating a lunch-only or dinner-only pattern have the same level of weight loss. Once again, stay tuned!

Tip 3: Count Your Calories—Not!

One of the wonderful features of the Every-Other-Day Diet is that it's incredibly easy to follow: all you do is eat 500 calories on Diet Day and whatever you want on Feast Day. I've never talked to a single person who really likes calorie counting, even with the new smartphone apps that make the process a little easier, like Lose It! or MyFitness Pal.

Counting calories makes it seem like a calculator is a utensil you have to use at every meal, like mealtime is a contest where you're both competitor and scorekeeper, and you're always about to be (and feel) defeated. In short, it's an annoying mealtime chore you'd rather not do. You want to *enjoy* food, not tabulate it.

Well, the recipes and guidance in this book guarantee that you'll never have to do any complex calorie counting while you're on the Every-Other-Day Diet. Because we've done all the counting for you, in advance.

There are typically two times you take in calories on Diet Day: at your lunch or dinner (about 400 calories), and when you eat your snack (about 100 calories). And there are two ways you can go about your Diet Day meals.

You can make your own food, in which case chapter 4 will be hugely helpful. It provides 28 days of 400-calorie lunches, 28 days of 400-calorie dinners, and 28 days of 100-calorie snacks—and those 84 recipes can provides *months* of easeful Diet Days.

Say, for example, that your New Year's resolution is to lose 20 pounds, and you start the Every-Other-Day Diet on January 2. In January, you'll have 15 Diet Days; in February, you'll have 14. If you choose lunch as your Diet Day meal, the lunch recipes in chapter 4 will guide you through two months of dieting. If you decide to switch to dinner for Diet Days in March and April, the recipes will guide you through nearly two more months of Diet Days.

In other words, there are enough recipes in chapter 4 for nearly *four months* of Diet Days, without ever having to count a single calorie or eat the same recipe twice. And because those recipes are simple (no recipe has more than seven ingredients); speedy (cooking and preparation times are always under 30 minutes); and tasty, you're in for a couple of months of easeful (and even fun) Diet Days.

Or you can always opt to microwave an entrée from chapter 5. Many of today's frozen entrées are twenty-first-century wonders of culinary ingenuity, delivering maximum flavor and nutrition. They're also perfect for super-easy EOD dieting, since the label tells you exactly how many calories they contain. In chapter 5, we've listed dozens of frozen entrées that are 400 calories or less. And we've provided the Two-Month Diet Day Meal Plan, which organizes the entrées into a varied and appetizing pace of Diet Day meals. If you want to diet for longer than two months on frozen entrées, just repeat the plan.

Many participants in my studies prefer the ease and simplicity of using frozen entrées for their Diet Day meal, and you might feel the same way. You won't have to think twice (or even once) about calories, and preparation takes hardly any time at all.

Tip 4: Make a Plan for the Day—and Stick with It

What's the biggest mistake my study participants made on Diet Day? Not knowing *exactly* what they were going to eat when mealtime rolled around. Because if you're hungry, you're likely to eat more than 500 calories.

There's an easy way to avoid that mistake: choose your lunch or dinner (and snack) for Diet Day the *night before* and rest easy that you'll have a very successful Diet Day tomorrow.

Tip 5: Don't Eat Mini-Meals

Over my years of research into EOD dieting, I've been asked by many study participants if they could divide the calories of their Diet Day meal into several low-calorie mini-meals. That way, they reasoned, they could eat throughout the day and feel less hungry. My answer is always *no*. And I have a very good reason for saying no: I want my study participants to actually lose weight!

The problem with eating mini-meals on Diet Day—for example, three 150-calorie meals—is that most of us tend to underestimate calories. What you *think* is 150 calories is probably 200, 250, or more. So instead of eating the 400-calorie Diet Day meal and a 100-calorie Diet Day snack, you might eat three mini-meals of 200, 250, or 300 calories, eat a lot more than 500 calories on Diet Day, and slow the pace and amount of weight loss. But if you eat only one meal a day, you have only one opportunity to miscalculate calories. And if you do err one time a day—maybe consuming 100 excess calories—it's not such a big deal.

However, there's an exception to this rule. When you prepare and eat a lunch or dinner recipe from chapter 4, or a frozen entrée from chapter 5, you know the *exact* amount of calories you're consuming because we've totaled the calories in the recipe, or they're right there on the label of the frozen foods or packaged snacks. So feel free to eat the meal any way you like: all at once; half for lunch and half for dinner; or even in thirds. I don't think this strategy is ideal, because it doesn't reflect what worked in my studies. But if you're absolutely certain your intake is under 500 calories, you're still on the Every-Other-Day Diet.

PROTEIN PACKS A PUNCH

Protein is a powerful tool to fight off hunger and keep you feeling full longer. Researchers at the University of Missouri divided 27 overweight men on a calorie-restricted diet into high- or normal-protein groups. The high-protein group felt *twice* as full during the day as the normal-protein group. "These data support the consumption of high protein intake, but not greater eating frequency, for improved appetite control and satiety [fullness]...during calorie restriction-induced weight loss," the researchers concluded.[6]

In a similar study from researchers at the University of Kansas Medical Center, also published in *Obesity*, 13 obese people ate either three or six meals a day, and the meals were either normal or high protein.[7] And once again, eating more frequently didn't reduce the participants' hunger—but eating protein did. In fact, eating six meals a day led to "lower daily fullness"; the folks who ate *more* frequently felt *more* hungry throughout the day.

Bottom line: Protein is crucial for helping you feel full and staving off hunger. The hunger-taming power of protein is why many of the recipes in chapter 4, like the Turkey and Avocado Sandwich, and many of the frozen foods in chapter 5, like Pepperoni Pizza, have plenty of protein.

A final note: Don't look to protein bars to mute your appetite. Not only are they typically too high in calories for the Every-Other-Day Diet, but they're often artificially sweetened, which can stimulate appetite. You'll read more about the downsides of artificial sweeteners later in this chapter.

PAUL'S STORY: "I FOUND ALTERNATE-DAY FASTING INCREDIBLY EASY TO DO."

Weight loss: 49 pounds

Paul Gower is a 52-year-old in the Fire Safety Department in Malvern, Worcestershire, in England. On Diet Day, he limits his intake to several cups of beef broth, water, four or five cups of coffee, and some raw vegetables, like celery sticks. "If I eat more than that I find it quite difficult to stop eating," he told us. But that approach to Diet Day has

(continued)

definitely worked for him. In August 2012, when he started every-other-day dieting, the 5'11" Gower weighed 231 pounds. After a year on the diet, he weighs 182.

"I found alternate-day fasting incredibly easy to do," he said. "The hardest part of the diet is that I do the majority of cooking for my family—I've always cooked and I love to cook. In the early days, I would serve the meal and walk away. Now, I just sit with them and drink my beef broth and eat my celery sticks, and I can cope with it."

In fact, Diet Days are so easy he barely thinks about them. "I'm hardly aware of them, they're so much a part of my routine," he said. "And I know that I can always eat whatever I want tomorrow—and I do! I've tried many other diets over the years and this is the one that works for me."

Tip 6: Don't Skimp on the Fat

Most diets require you to change not only the *amount* of food you're eating, but also the *type* of food. If you're on a Paleo Diet, you can't eat grains, beans, or dairy products. If you're on Atkins, you cut carbs. With a plant-based or vegan diet, red meat, fish, dairy, and eggs are forbidden. If you're on the Ornish Diet, you restrict fat. If you've decided to hang out in The Zone, you juggle macronutrients, carefully calibrating every meal to include 40% "good" carbs, 30% fat, and 30% protein. And the latest fashion in dieting—reflected in plans like the 17-Day Diet and the Dukan Diet—restricts foods in complex stages, phases, and cycles that require a complete change in eating habits every few weeks.

The Every-Other-Day Diet *doesn't* make complicated dietary demands. On Diet Day, you can stick with your current pattern of eating, whatever it is. You don't have to restock your refrigerator and pantry and eat in ways you've never eaten before. Diet Day is about eating fewer *calories*—not some strange mix of macronutrients, or a confusing menu of "allowed" and "forbidden" foods.

Bottom line: You can eat anything you want on Diet Day—as long as you eat only 500 calories. And by anything, I mean *anything*—including high-fat foods.

I don't like to see EOD dieters suffer from the problem my coauthor Bill and I have dubbed *lipidophobia*: fear of dietary fat. In fact, I'd like to *encourage* you to eat high-fat foods on Diet Day. I know that sounds like weight-loss heresy. But it's the *proven* approach to maximizing success on the EOD diet. You'll recall from chapter 1, some of my studies have explored whether eating high- or low-fat food on Diet Day plays any role in how much weight you lose. In one of those studies, I divided participants into two groups: one group ate high-fat foods on Diet Day and the other ate low-fat foods. The folks on the high-fat diet (45% fat, 15% protein, 40% carbohydrates) had the following results:

- They lost 17% more weight.
- They lost 32% more body fat.
- They had an 8% increase in muscle (lean body mass), while the low-fat group had no increase.

I had a theory about the pound-shedding, fat-shedding power of high fat: I thought the low-fat group felt deprived and cheated on Diet Day. And when my colleagues and I analyzed the data, we found out that was the case; the folks eating low-fat foods on Diet Day cheated nearly *twice* as often as the folks eating high-fat foods.

So go ahead and enjoy high-fat foods—both on Diet Day and on Feast Day. They're delicious and satisfying and, as research suggests, even good for you! Below are some examples of high-fat foods and their benefits.

More fish oil, longer life. A study from researchers at the Harvard School of Public Health found that older people with high blood levels of omega-3 fatty acids—the DHA (docosahexaenoic acid) and EPA (eicosapentaenoic acid) primarily found in fish oil—had a 27% lower risk of death from any cause, mostly because fewer of them died from heart disease, which kills so many people.[8] In fact, people with the highest blood levels of omega-3 fats at age 65 lived an average of 2.2 years longer than people with the lowest levels. Yet many of the adherents of low-fat, plant-based diets specifically tell you *not* to eat EPA- and DHA-rich fatty fish.

Olive oil and nuts—two high-fat foods—prevent heart attack and stroke. In a study published in the *New England Journal of Medicine*, Spanish researchers divided more than 7,000 people at high risk for heart disease into three groups: two groups ate a Mediterranean diet rich in either olive oil or nuts. The fat-rich diets lowered the risk of heart attack, stroke, and death from heart disease by 30% compared to a low-fat diet—a benefit so impressive the researchers stopped the study, because they couldn't ethically keep the third group on a diet that didn't include high-fat foods.[9]

Saturated fat doesn't cause heart disease. Saturated fat is found mainly in meat and dairy products, and we've been told again and again that it trashes our arteries, triggering heart attacks and strokes, and that everybody should eat less. Is that good advice? Not according to a study from scientists at the Oakland Research Institute in California, published in the *American Journal of Clinical Nutrition*.[10] The researchers analyzed data from 21 other studies, involving more than 340,000 people. They found "no significant evidence for concluding that dietary saturated fat is associated with increased risk of coronary heart disease or cardiovascular disease."

On a smaller scale, several of my studies have shown that people who ate high-fat foods on Diet Day had improvements in their risk factors for cardiovascular disease that matched the improvements in people who ate low-fat foods. In other words, high-fat wasn't hurting them, but weight loss was helping them!

It's high time we stop being afraid of high-fat foods; that's why they're an enjoyable element of the Every-Other-Day Diet.

GERD'S STORY: "I'M 51 YEARS OLD—BUT I FEEL LIKE I'M 30."

Weight loss: 21 pounds

At 6'3", 51-year-old Gerd Eichele can still carry his weight quite well. "I'm a big guy, with big bones," he told us. But a couple of years ago he realized he was carrying a little too much weight. "A friend of mine took my picture and when I saw it I was shocked. I thought, 'Whoa, look at that gut!'"

(continued)

Gerd started on a program of alternate-day fasting in September 2011. He kept his caloric intake on Diet Day at around 750 calories, eating two very low-calorie meals a day and one snack. A breakfast would typically be a medium-sized bowl of oatmeal, a boiled egg, and a glass of orange juice. He would snack on an apple during the day and have a bag of quick-cook steamed vegetables for dinner. When he started every-other-day fasting he weighed 239 pounds. Today he weighs 218.

"A lot of people started commenting on my weight—even my in-laws. Alternate-day fasting was a little tough at first," he said. "But once I got into the swing of it, it was easy. What surprises me the most is that when I wake up in the morning after a day of fasting I'm not really all that hungry."

Gerd attributes his weight loss not only to every-other-day dieting, but to drinking *lots* of water, which helps him feel full during the day. "I drink a liter [34 ounces] of water right after I get up in the morning, and continue to drink water throughout the day," he said.

His third weight-loss secret, along with every-other-day dieting and water: regular exercise. "I walk about three miles a day, and six or seven miles once a week," he said. "I listen to music or podcasts while I walk, and the time really flies by. This combination—every-other-day fasting, lots of water, and regular exercise—really hit the mark."

Gerd feels like he could lose a few more pounds and "discover" his abs, which are still covered up by a bit of fat. "I'm sure that with alternate-day fasting, drinking plenty of water, and regular exercise I'll reach that goal, too."

Tip 7: If You're Eating Out on Diet Day, Check the Menu Before You Go!

Of course, at some point, you're going to find yourself eating out on Diet Day, which is a little bit like tiptoeing through a minefield where the mines are calories that could blow up your diet. It's risky! For that reason, I strongly recommend you try to avoid it as much as possible, but if you do eat out, here is my top tip: plan ahead.

If you're going to eat out at a fast-food restaurant like McDonald's or Burger King or a casual-dining restaurant like Applebee's, Friday's, or Chili's, before you go, go online and check the calorie counts of items on the menu that you like, to see what's a match for the calorie limit of Diet Day.

For example, Applebee's lists some entrées as under 550 calories, not bad for your meal on Diet Day (if you haven't had a snack). They include the Roast Garlic Sirloin, the Napa Chicken and Portobellos, and Zesty Roma Chicken and Shrimp. Other entrées are endorsed by Weight Watchers.

You can assume that just about everything else on the menu—*including the appetizers*—is over 500 calories. Way over. For example, open the "Nutritional Info" PDF at the Applebee's site (www.applebees.com), and you'll discover that many appetizers are 1,200 or more calories—and not a single appetizer is even close to 500 calories. Have a bowl of Baked Potato Soup—a dish you might assume is relatively low-calorie—and you've downed 470 calories. The Green Goddess Wedge Salad is 560 calories. I'm not criticizing Applebee's; I'm just using it as an example to show you how tricky it is to eat out on Diet Day.

My essential message is this: *Know* the calories in any dish you're ordering by first finding out the calorie level online. And *don't* order any dish or meal if you're guessing its calorie level. Chances are, you're guessing wrong.

When it comes to fast-food restaurants, the number of meals that can work on Diet Day may surprise you. For example, McDonald's claims that 80% of the items on its menu are under 400 calories—a good fit for Diet Day. And their claim is true. A Filet-O-Fish is 390 calories. A Cheeseburger is 300 calories. Six Chicken McNuggets are 280 calories. And a Premium Caesar Salad with Grilled Chicken is 190 calories.

So if you're determined to eat at McDonald's on Diet Day (or at any other fast-food restaurant), you McCan! Just go online *first*, figure out what you want, check the calories, and stick to your calorie-smart choices when you're at the restaurant.

Tip 8: Make the Most of Your Snack on Diet Day

The typical Diet Day includes a 400-calorie meal (either lunch or dinner) and a 100-calorie snack. If you eat a Diet Day lunch or dinner that is *less* than 400 calories, you can eat a snack that is *more* than 100 calories. Or if you choose a frozen entrée that is around 300 calories—and there are many such entrées in the meal plan in chapter 5—you can eat two 100-calorie snacks.

What kind of snack should you eat? In chapter 4, you'll find delicious recipes for twenty-eight 100-calorie snacks, like Berry Smoothie Pops, Greek Yogurt Parfait, and Chocolate Stack. In chapter 5, you'll find an extensive list of packaged snack foods that range from 50 to 160 calories, supplementing the calories in your lunch or dinner entrée on Diet Day to add up to 500 calories for the day.

When should you have your snack? The participants in my studies have eaten their Diet Day snack any time of day (or night): first thing in the morning, midmorning, midafternoon, early evening, before bed—even in the middle of the night! What's best is what's best for *you*—eat your snack when you want it the most and enjoy it the most.

During the first two weeks or so of the EOD Diet—when you're still feeling hungry on Diet Day—eat your snack at the time of day you're hungriest. In other words, use it to reduce hunger. After two weeks on the Every-Other-Day Diet, when hunger on Diet Day has pretty much disappeared, eat the snack for enjoyment and energy, at the time of day when you find you're most refreshed and renewed by having something to eat.

Aside from your personal preferences, nutritional science provides a few guidelines about the best time of day to snack for weight loss.

Afternoon is better than midmorning. Researchers at the University of Illinois studied 123 overweight women who were in a one-year weight-loss program. Those who snacked in the afternoon lost 7% more weight than those who snacked midmorning, the researchers reported in the *Journal of the American Dietetic Association*.[11]

Nighttime might not be the right time. Women who snacked at night burned 12% less fat than people who snacked during the daytime, reported Japanese researchers. "Eating at night...increases the risk of obesity," they wrote in the *American Journal of Physiology: Regulatory, Integrative and Comparative Physiology*.[12]

SCIENTIFIC SURPRISE: SNACKING CAN BE GOOD FOR YOU

Americans are snacking more than ever: over the past few decades, the percentage of American adults who snack rose from 71% to 97%. We're eating an average of one more snack per day than we used to. The percentage of total daily calories from snacks rose from 18% to 24%. And we're consuming more salty snacks, cookies, candy, and sugar-sweetened beverages. There are plenty of studies that link snacking—and its added calories—to added pounds. But what you typically don't hear is the *good* news about snacking. For example:

If you start eating smaller, low-calorie snacks, you quickly adapt to the smaller size and regularly eat smaller snacks. Researchers at the Center for Human Nutrition at the University of Colorado studied 59 people, testing the effect of eating 100-calorie snacks. They found the individuals quickly adapted to the smaller snacks and stopped eating bigger snacks.[13]

Well, you won't find any snack larger than 160 calories in chapters 4 and 5 (and most are 100 calories), but you'll quickly get used to eating and enjoying these smaller, lower-calorie snacks. Bon appétidbit!

Snacks improve your diet. A team of researchers from Auburn University in Alabama noted that snacking has a bad rap: it's thought to contribute nothing more than empty calories to the diet. But in a five-year study of more than 11,000 adults, they found ("contrary to expectation") that folks who snacked scored *higher* on the Healthy Eating Index. The more people snacked, the more fruits, whole grains, and milk products they ate. "Snacking was associated with a more nutrient-dense diet," wrote the researchers in the *Journal of the Academy of Nutrition and Dietetics.*[14]

Seniors—start your snacking! When the researchers at Auburn focused on 2,000 people age 65 and older, they found those who snacked more also had higher intakes of vitamins A, C, E, and beta-carotene, and the minerals magnesium and potassium. "Nutritional benefits obtained from snack food and beverages warrant their inclusion in older adults' diet," they concluded in the *Journal of the American Dietetic Association.*[15]

Snacks help you maintain weight loss. In a study of 257 adults, people who lost weight and maintained it ate 21% more snacks than people who were overweight. "Two snacks per day may be important in weight loss maintenance," wrote the researchers in the *Journal of the American Dietetic Association.*[16]

Bottom line: Develop a knack for snacks!

THE FOUR BEST WAYS TO EASE YOUR HUNGER ON DIET DAY

My research shows that people feel hungry on Diet Day for about the first two to three weeks of the Every-Other-Day Diet, and then hunger pretty much disappears. How do you deal with your hunger on Diet Day during those first few weeks? EOD dieters say a couple of strategies work best.

1. Drink a Glass (or Two) of Water

The folks in my studies consistently tell me that when they're hungry on Diet Day, nothing works as well to mute their appetite as drinking a glass (or two) of water. They drink 8, 10, 12, or 16 ounces, and in just a few minutes their hunger level noticeably declines.

These EOD dieters are finding out for themselves what scientists have been discovering over the past couple of years: study after study is showing the power of water to diminish appetite.

Here are some of the recent findings supporting the power of a glass of water to wash away Diet Day discomfort and help you shed pounds.

Drink water before a meal and feel fuller and less hungry. Researchers at Virginia Tech studied 50 people, dividing them into two groups: half drank 17 ounces (one-half liter) of water 30 minutes before lunch, and half didn't. Those who drank water ate an average of 58 fewer calories at lunchtime and also felt less hungry and more full.[17]

In a similar study from the same researchers, people who drank a half liter of water 30 minutes before breakfast ate 74 fewer calories in the meal.[18]

"Drinking water reduces sensations of hunger and increases satiety, the sensation of feeling full," says Brenda Davy, PhD, RD, the leader of these studies and an associate professor in the Department of Nutrition, Foods and Exercise at Virginia Tech.

Drink more water, burn more calories. Drinking one-half liter of water triggers the body to increase calorie burning by 24% over the next hour, reported German researchers in the *Journal of Clinical Endocrinology and Metabolism*.[19]

These researchers aren't talking about drinking a glass of *cold* water, thereby speeding up metabolism as your body tries to reheat itself. *Any* temperature of drinking water causes an increase in calorie-burning, because a glass of water stimulates the sympathetic nervous system, increasing metabolic rate.

Drink more water, lose more weight. Researchers at Virginia Tech studied 40 people: 20 were instructed to drink 16 ounces of water before every meal and record their daily water intake; the other 20 didn't pay any extra attention to their daily hydration. After one year, the group that was attentive to water intake lost 87% more weight.[20]

Bottom line: Hydrate! Drink 16 ounces (2 cups) of water *whenever* you feel hungry, 30 minutes or so before your Diet Day meal, and 30 minutes or so before your Diet Day snack. Another good strategy: carry a water bottle with you and drink as often as possible throughout the day.

SICK OF PLAIN WATER? INFUSE!

Many of the participants in my studies said they got tired of drinking plain water and solved the problem by drinking carbonated or seltzer water, or adding a spritz of lemon or lime. But there's another way to spruce up a plain glass of water, turning it into a delicious, delicately flavored drink: infusion.

You can buy an "infusion pitcher" for $15 to $25 at Bed Bath & Beyond, Target, Costco, and many other retail and

---

(continued)

online stores. Essentially, it's a big water pitcher with a rod or chamber in the middle, into which you can put, well, just about *anything* you like. The infusing ingredient stays in the chamber and flavors the water. Try lemon, orange and/or grapefruit slices, berries or cherries, cucumbers and lemongrass (the combo used in many spas). Watermelon and kiwi. Or use herbs like mint, rosemary, lavender, or chamomile to make a delicious iced tea. Really, any combination of fruits, herbs, or refreshing vegetables you'd like to try. And you can use any type of water—plain, carbonated, or seltzer. The infusion ingredients will stay fresh for 10 days, as long as you refrigerate the pitcher. Just refill and drink up!

2. Skip the Diet Soda and Avoid Artificial Sweeteners— They Might Make You *Hungrier*

Because water is so effective at reducing hunger and aiding weight loss, you might think *any* no-calorie beverage can do the same, like no-calorie diet sodas, diet energy drinks, and diet sports drinks. These artificially sweetened beverages can be a good strategy for some people, but I'm not a big fan of drinking diet sodas or other artificially sweetened beverages on Diet Day, for a few reasons:

More diet sodas result in more eating. A study in the journal *Appetite* showed that people who drink two or more artificially sweetened drinks per day have a *harder* time controlling their appetite and have a tendency to overeat.[21] And scientists think they may know why. Researchers in the Department of Psychiatry at Yale University School of Medicine scanned the brains of 26 people while they used an artificial sweetener and found that being exposed to a sweet taste *without* ingesting any calories may cause the brain to generate cravings for more sweet foods! I'm not surprised by these results. In my studies, about 4 out of 5 participants get a surge of hunger after drinking a diet soda.

Drinking three diet sodas a day doubles your risk of obesity. In a seven-year study from the University of Texas Health Science Center involving more than 3,600 people, those who drank three or more artificially sweetened beverages per day were nearly *twice* as likely to become overweight or obese. "These findings raise the question," wrote the researchers in *Obesity*, whether artificially sweetened beverages "might be fueling—rather than fighting—our escalating obesity epidemic."[22]

Artificial sweeteners can lead to disease. Other studies link diet sodas to disease. Compared to people who don't drink diet soda, those who drink diet soda had

- *a 16% higher risk of stroke*, per diet soda, per day. (In other words, if you regularly drink two diet sodas per day, your risk is 32% higher.[23])
- *a 42% higher risk of leukemia,* per diet soda per day.[24]
- *a 67% higher risk for type 2 diabetes*, from daily consumption of one or more diet sodas. Research published in *Diabetes Care* shows that diet soda stimulates the release of GLP-1 (glucagon-like peptide 1), a compound linked to the development of type 2 diabetes.[25]
- *a 220% higher risk for chronic kidney disease* for people consuming two or more diet sodas per day.[26]

So my advice is to limit artificial sweeteners wherever you can. However, if occasionally you want to drink beverages with a no-calorie sweetener, I recommend ones with either saccharin (like Sweet 'N Low), which has a long record of safety; or stevia, made from the leaves of the stevia plant, a sweet-tasting herb in the chrysanthemum family.

A health professional whom Bill interviews regularly asked his staff to conduct a taste test of stevia products; they picked Body Ecology and SweetLeaf as the best-tasting brands. Bill's wife, who uses stevia exclusively as a sweetener, favors NuNaturals' NuStevia. Many other people choose the popular brands Pure Via and Truvía. And there are many others. Try different brands and see which one tastes best to you.

Why don't we recommend aspartame (Equal; NutraSweet) or sucralose (Splenda)? Because those are the two sweeteners used in most diet sodas, beverages increasingly linked to health problems, as we just discussed. As we were writing this book, a new study in *Diabetes Care* from researchers at the University of Washington in Seattle showed that ingesting Splenda spiked blood sugar and insulin levels in obese people.[27]

CAN YOU DRINK ALCOHOL ON DIET DAY?

For many of us, drinking a beer, a glass of wine, or a cocktail is one of the happy pleasures of daily life—it refreshes, relaxes, and enhances your enjoyment of social time with family and friends. Research also shows that moderate drinking—no more than two drinks a day for men and one drink a day for women—can reduce the risk of heart disease. (One drink is 5 ounces of wine, 12 ounces of beer, or 1½ ounces of distilled spirits or liquor, such as whiskey or vodka.)

If you enjoy alcohol in moderation, there's no need to stop on the Every-Other-Day Diet. Like any other food or beverage, there's no limit to alcohol intake on Feast Day, other than common sense.

But what about Diet Day? Well, think carefully before imbibing. Because along with that pleasant buzz, alcohol can deliver a lot of calories.

For example, if you down an 8-ounce margarita, you're also downing nearly 300 calories—60% of your Diet Day quota! A White Russian (the favored drink of The Dude, the chubby star of the movie *The Big Lebowski*) delivers a whopping 425 calories—basically, your *meal* on Diet Day.

Not all drinks are super-caloric, of course. Red wine delivers 110 calories; beer, 150 to 200. There are ultra-light beers that deliver less than 100 calories. And you don't have to down an entire drink: for example, if you limit a glass of white wine to 4 ounces, it's about 90 calories.

My recommendation for drinking an alcoholic beverage on Diet Day is simple: Just say no. They're too high in calories. And because they affect your judgment and are a typical mealtime accompaniment, it's too easy to decide to have a second drink. Before you know it, Diet Day has turned into eat, drink, and be merry day.

If you do decide to have a drink on Diet Day, have only one, and consider it your snack for the day, consuming a

(continued)

beverage that matches the calorie level of your lunch or din-ner. If your entrée is 350 calories, you could accompany it with a 150-calorie beer.

Bottom line: If you'd like to "snack" on an alcoholic bev-erage on Diet Day, go ahead. But be aware of the calories the drink contains, and don't overdo it.

3. A Cup of Joe or Tea a Day Can Keep the Hunger Away

A cup of black coffee or a cup of tea are both good ways to cut hunger without adding calories. And they both have their own hunger-controlling, weight-busting benefits. When overweight and obese people drank a cup of strong coffee with breakfast, they ate less at lunch and throughout the day, reported researchers in *Obesity*.[28]

More coffee, more weight loss. In a 12-year study of nearly 58,000 people, those who increased their coffee con-sumption during the study gained less weight, reported researchers from the Harvard School of Public Health.[29] When researchers analyzed 11 studies on green tea and dieting, they similarly found that people who drank tea lost up to 3.3 more pounds than people who didn't.

Catechins and caffeine: low hunger, high fullness. Bill's book *The Natural Fat-Loss Pharmacy* devotes an entire chapter to the appetite-taming, pound-preventing power of tea—black, green, and white (oolong) tea—with green tea leading the way. The secret ingredient in tea: *catechins*, pow-erful plant compounds with a wide range of health-giving effects, like lowering the risk of heart disease and cancer.

A beverage containing green tea catechins and caffeine (along with fiber) "created the lowest hunger and the highest fullness ratings and the lowest energy [calorie] intake at the next meal," reported researchers in the journal *Appetite*.[30]

Tea trims body fat. Habitual tea drinkers (15 ounces daily) have 20% less body fat than people who don't drink tea, according to a study in *Obesity Research*.

Catechins help people burn more calories and fat. Drinking a catechin-rich tea throughout the day triggered 12% more fat-burning than drinking water, according to a study in the *Journal of Nutrition*. In another study, obese dieters who took a supplement with green tea catechins burned 43 more calories per day—and lost 7.3 more pounds after 12 weeks, compared to dieters who didn't take the green tea supplement.

Catechins help you do better weight maintenance. Getting more green tea catechins in the diet helped people "significantly maintain body weight after a period of weight loss," reported Dutch researchers in the *International Journal of Obesity*.[31]

Bottom line: Coffee and/or tea, particularly green tea, are great choices for no-calorie drinks on Diet Day. And they're good for you, too. Recent studies link regular coffee drinking to a wide range of health benefits, including less risk of type 2 diabetes, gallbladder disease, Alzheimer's disease, Parkinson's disease, and liver cancer. One 13-year study of more than 52,000 people showed that regular coffee drinkers even had lower "all-cause mortality"—during the study, they died less frequently from any cause, compared to people who didn't drink coffee.[32]

Green tea also has a positive effect on health: studies link green tea and its catechins to lower risk for heart disease, and lower risk for many types of cancer, type 2 diabetes, and Alzheimer's disease.

But take care with the cream and sugar. If you want to add a little milk and sugar to your coffee or tea, go right ahead, but you'll have to count calories. For example, a tablespoon of skim milk has 6 calories; a tablespoon of whole milk, 9; and a tablespoon of half-and-half, 20. A packet of sugar adds 11 calories. If you have four cups of coffee on Diet Day with a touch of whole milk and a packet of sugar, you're adding 80 calories—in effect, your four cups of coffee have become your daily snack.

4. Chew Up Your Hunger with Sugar-Free Gum

One of the best ways to stave off hunger on Diet Day, say my study participants, is to *chew gum.* It keeps your mouth busy. And it seems to "fool" your body into thinking you're eating something. Check out these studies about the effects of gum chewing:

People feel less hungry and burn more calories. In his book *Breakthroughs in Natural Healing 2011*, Bill reported on two studies showing that chewing sugar-free gum can help you feel less hungry, so you eat fewer calories and burn more. The first study was conducted by Kathleen Melanson, PhD, RD, an associate professor of nutrition and food science at the University of Rhode Island. The 35 participants in the two-day study chewed sugar-free gum on only one of the two days in three 20-minute sessions of "relaxed, natural" chewing: one session before breakfast, and two sessions between breakfast and lunch. The results? On the day of gum-chewing, participants felt less hungry, consumed an average of 68 fewer calories at lunch, and didn't consume more calories later in the day. The participants also burned about 5% more calories during the gum-chewing sessions. And they felt more upbeat on the day they chewed gum: they had more energy, and it seemed to take less energy to accomplish tasks.

"Gum chewing may be a useful addition to a weight-management program," concluded Dr. Melanson, who reported her research at an annual meeting of the Obesity Society. "Gum-chewing might cut hunger and calorie intake in two ways," Dr. Melanson told Bill. "The sensations in the mouth might send 'I'm full' signals to the brain's appetite center. And nerves in the muscles of the jaw that are stimulated by gum chewing might send those signals, too.

"If you're attempting to lose weight, give gum-chewing a try to see if it works to help you feel less hungry and cut calories," she continued. "Use sugar-free gum as one tool in your weight-loss toolbox."

Seven smart times to chew gum. Another study on gum-chewing in overweight people was reported at the same meeting by Leah Whigham, PhD, a nutrition scientist at the government's Grand Forks Human Nutrition Research Center in North Dakota.

Dr. Whigham and her colleagues found that overweight people who typically needed a lot of "cognitive restraint" in order to control their eating habits—people who had to remind themselves again and again *not* to eat, so they wouldn't mindlessly snack or eat when they weren't hungry—ate fewer daily calories when they chewed gum six times a day for 15 minutes each time.

Dr. Whigham suggests chewing sugar-free gum at the following times:

- when you're craving a high-calorie snack
- when watching TV, instead of snacking
- for 15 minutes immediately after lunch or dinner
- when you go out to eat, while waiting for the main course
- in "high-risk" situations for overeating, such as at parties, weddings, sporting events, or the movies
- when you're bored, since boredom is often a trigger for eating and overeating
- when you're stressed, since stress is also a trigger

More gum-chewing, less hunger, less appetite, and less craving for sweets. In a four-day study, researchers in England asked 60 people to eat lunch and then rate their hunger, appetite, and craving for sweet and salty snacks every hour for three hours. On two days of the study, the participants chewed gum for 15 minutes every hour, for a total of 45 minutes of chewing over the three hours. On the other two days, they didn't chew gum. "Chewing gum for at least 45 minutes significantly suppressed hunger, appetite and craving for snacks and promoted fullness," wrote the researchers in *Appetite*.[33] "This study," they continued, demonstrated the "benefit of chewing gum…to those seeking an aid to appetite control."

More chewing, less stress. Chewing gum can also help

you resist stress. In a study conducted by researchers in the United Kingdom, people who chewed gum daily for two weeks had less "perceived stress" and felt they could get more work done, compared to people who didn't chew gum.[34]

In a similar study, in *Current Medical Research and Opinion*, people said that stressful emotions (not feeling relaxed, feeling tense) increased when they *didn't* chew gum.[35]

And in a study by Australian researchers, chewing gum reduced anxiety and stress, reduced the production of the stress hormone cortisol, and increased alertness.[36]

EXERCISE IS OKAY ON DIET DAY IF YOU EXERCISE BEFORE A MEAL

As you read in chapter 1, I've conducted studies to determine if people could exercise comfortably on the EOD Diet. The results: study participants exercised without problems, whether they worked out on Diet Day, Feast Day, or on both. But there was one caveat: Exercising late in the day on Diet Day wasn't a good idea. People who tried to do so felt ravenous after their workout, but they'd already consumed 400 of their 500 daily calories, or all 500.

There are three good times to exercise on Diet Day:

- first thing in the morning, perhaps eating your 100-calorie snack right afterward; or
- right before lunch; or
- right before dinner, if you chose dinner as your Diet Day meal

In other words, exercise *before* a meal.

You'll find much more about EOD dieting and exercise in chapter 6, "Every-Other-Day Dieting and Exercise."

SARAH'S STORY: "I WAS A SIZE 18 AND NOW I'M A 12."

Weight loss: 36 pounds

Sarah is a nurse who works at the Veterans Administration hospital near the University of Illinois-Chicago, where she saw a flyer recruiting people for a weight-loss study using alternate-day modified fasting. "I needed to lose weight, and I thought participating in the study would be a great way to do it," she said.

And lose weight she did. At 5'2" tall, Sarah started the diet weighing 207 pounds, and now she weighs 171.

"I've gone down six dress sizes!" she exclaimed. "And my cholesterol dropped, too—from slightly over 200 to 180. The first two weeks of the Every-Other-Day Diet were kind of rough, because of the hunger on Diet Day, but that went away, and every-other-day dieting became my life. And it was *easy*. For example, if I knew a special occasion was coming up on a Diet Day, I'd just flip-flop a Feast Day and a Diet Day. The key was *planning*.

"I also found that I ate much less on Feast Day than I thought I would. After a few weeks on the diet, it seemed like I was satisfied more quickly by my Feast Day meals, and I almost never overate."

Sarah also added exercise to her regimen. "Along with the EOD Diet, I do water aerobics, kick-boxing, jogging, walking—anything to help me burn more calories and look thinner," she said. "I also weigh myself regularly, to make sure I'm not gaining the weight back."

DON'T WORRY ABOUT CHEATING NOW AND THEN

Let's face it: you're probably going to cheat now and then. You're only human!

So, don't worry about it! The participants in my studies who lose the most weight are "adherent" on Diet Day (that is, they don't cheat) on 8 or 9 days out of 10. In other words, they occasionally cheat—and it's no big deal. After all, sometimes your Diet Day is going to fall on a special occasion, like a holiday, birthday party, or another time when you want to join in the fun.

Go ahead and do it! For example, if Diet Day falls on Thanksgiving, eat Thanksgiving dinner, even if the day before Thanksgiving was a Feast Day. The day *after* Thanksgiving can be Diet Day.

It's fine if once or twice a month Diet Day doesn't work out. If you eat 500 calories on 8 or 9 out of 10 Diet Days, you *will* lose weight. The trick is, if you go off the EOD Diet, just go back on it again the next Diet Day. Cheat on Tuesday; get back on the diet on Thursday. Another possible strategy: if you blow it on Diet Day, relax, turn it into Feast Day, and do Diet Day tomorrow. But...

Don't beat yourself up—you're just hurting yourself.

Don't feel like a failure—you're on the science-proven way to weight-loss success!

Don't binge if you go off the diet on Diet Day—because you can eat whatever you want (and as much as you want) on Feast Day.

Relax—and just go back on the diet.

THE SIMPLEST DIET

The best feature of Diet Day is that it's so *easy*. You're not counting calories or following complex rules—you just eat one low-calorie meal and one snack. There are easy ways to tame Diet Day hunger, which only lasts for the first two weeks or so of the diet, after which you hardly notice it. And maybe the best feature of Diet Day is that it's followed by Feast Day, a day of unrestricted eating. Yes, a day of unlimited eating pleasure is actually part of a *diet*. To learn all about Feast Day, just turn the page.

EOD—EASY AS 1-2-3!

1. Follow one simple rule: eat 500 calories on Diet Day and eat whatever you want the next day.
2. Weigh yourself in the morning, make an eating plan for Diet Day, and eat a 400-calorie lunch or dinner and a 100-calorie snack.
3. Drink water, coffee, and/or tea, chew sugar-free gum, and use other easy methods to mute hunger on Diet Day.

CHAPTER 3

Feast Day

Eat all you want and anything you want—and keep losing weight!

This is the shortest chapter in the book, and for a good reason: there's only one easy-to-follow "rule" on Feast Day (the day that alternates with the 500-calorie modified fast of Diet Day). **Eat all the food you want, and eat any kind of food you want.**

I know, I know. It's hard to believe that you don't have to deprive yourself every day while dieting and that you can *still* lose weight; that a diet can contain a day on which you eat as much food as you want and whatever foods you want and you *still* lose weight. It probably goes against everything you've ever been told about dieting and everything you've ever done while on a diet.

Well, it also was hard to believe for some of my study participants. As veterans of many diets—and many days of diet-based deprivation and denial—they couldn't imagine how they could possibly lose weight while following the Feast Day "rule" every other day.

And because they so badly wanted to lose weight, many of them kept on restricting their food choices on Feast Day— until we talked them out of it! But once they got used to alternating a day of modified fasting with a day of unlimited eating, they loved it. Feast Day was a *relief* from restriction. And Feast Day made the 500 calories of Diet Day no big deal, because participants knew they could always eat their favorite foods tomorrow. Any food. In any quantity. At any time.

EOD DIETERS RAVE ABOUT FEAST DAY

Still find it hard to believe that you can eat whatever you want on Feast Day and lose weight? Then listen to what some veteran EOD dieters—people who have lost anywhere from 16 to 49 pounds—have to say about it:

I always enjoy Feast Day. "One day fasting and one day feasting is a wonderful pattern. Some days I eat a lot on my Feast Day, and some days I don't, but I always enjoy the day. And my weight continues to go down!" —*Paul, weight loss: 41 pounds*

I never feel deprived. "On the Every-Other-Day Diet, I can always eat the next day, so I never feel deprived. If I can't have it today, I can have it tomorrow. Knowing that, I can stay on the diet." —*Susan, weight loss: 42 pounds*

I stop eating when I feel satisfied and full. "At first, I really had a lot of anticipation about Feast Day, thinking I would just eat as much as I could. But when the day rolled around, I found myself thinking, 'Do I really need all that food?' I did eat a little more than normal, of course. But it seemed as if I was satisfied sooner at every meal—that I had learned what feeling *full* is all about, and I could stop eating when I felt full. If it wasn't for the Every-Other-Day Diet, I never would have learned how to do that." —*Sarah, weight loss: 17 pounds*

It's not difficult at all. "I eat heavy one day and light the next, and it's not difficult at all. It's become a habit." —*Bella, weight loss: 25 pounds*

I eat whenever I'm hungry. "On Feast Day, I'm very liberal about what I eat and don't eat. I start with a big, healthy breakfast, and then eat whenever I'm hungry, grazing throughout the day. I love it." —*Gerd, weight loss: 21 pounds*

I look forward to the days I'm not fasting. "I look forward to the days I'm not fasting and can do whatever I want. I don't have to think—'How many calories in this, how many calories in that?'—and that makes the day a whole lot easier." —*Victoria, weight loss: 27 pounds*

I've been on a lot of other diets, and I always get tired of them. "I like this diet because I get to *eat*. I've been on a lot of other diets—like diets where you drink two milkshakes and eat one meal a day—and I always get tired of them, because you're basically restricted to the same foods, over and over again." —*Andrea, weight loss: 16 pounds*

I eat what I want. "The Every-Other-Day Diet is very easy to do. I eat what I want on Feast Day, have one well-planned meal on Diet Day—and don't worry about it!" —*Paul, weight loss: 49 pounds*

Here's what's not hard to believe: Feast Day is the feature of the EOD Diet that study participants like the second best (right after losing all the weight they wanted to lose and keeping it off). And EOD dieters were delighted by the biggest surprise of every-other-day dieting: you don't lose control on Feast Day. You don't binge. You don't even eat all that much more. Remember, in my studies, EOD dieters ate only about 10% more calories than normal on Feast Day.

Do the pound-shedding math:

- You eat 25% of your normal calories on Diet Day.
- You eat 110% of your normal calories on Feast Day.
- Your two-day intake is an average of 67.5% of normal calories—32.5% below normal.
- And that lower level of calories drives steady, safe, *significant* weight loss.

The fact that folks don't go into overeating overdrive on Feast Day surprised me, too, at first. But after nearly a decade of research on hundreds of people, I feel confident that alternating a day of modified fasting with a day of unlimited eating *helps* overweight and obese people bring their appetite under control. Let's take a closer look at some of that research.

THE SURPRISING SCIENCE OF FEAST DAY

In our scientific studies on the EOD Diet, my colleagues and I take one of two approaches to providing food:

1. At the beginning of the study we teach the participants how to eat on Diet Day and Feast Day, and then the participants are on their own; or
2. we supply the participants with prepackaged, calorie-controlled meals and snacks for both Diet Day and Feast Day.

The first few studies we conducted followed Approach #2: the food was supplied. But we quickly found out (much to our amazement) that we were supplying *more* food on Feast Day than the study participants could eat.

Specifically, we gave study participants 125% of their normal caloric intake on Feast Day. But they always told us that we were giving them way too much food and they couldn't eat it all.

The same phenomenon is occurring in my three-year, NIH-sponsored study to test weight maintenance after the Every-Other-Day Diet. Once again, the study participants were given prepackaged, calorie-controlled meals—in this case, 50% of normal calories on Diet Day, and 150% on Feast Day.

Well, it turned out that nobody could eat all their "assigned" foods on Feast Day. Everybody in the study easily and spontaneously wanted to eat *less* than the 150%. It doesn't seem to make sense, right? After all, experts never tire of telling us that the main reason we Americans are overweight is the huge portions delivered by restaurants and convenience foods, and the 24/7 availability of food; that when a human being has access to a lot of food, a human being will *eat* a lot of food. So we imagine that people on the EOD Diet will inevitably pig out on Feast Day. And pork up. But they don't.

Feast Day isn't a trough. It's a fun, relaxed, and reasonable way to eat. After eating 25% of normal caloric intake on Diet Day, EOD dieters usually eat only 110% of normal calories on Feast Day. Below are my theories about why this happens.

Metabolic reboot. The EOD Diet may reset your metabolism—how your body uses food for energy—in ways that science doesn't yet understand but that are profoundly healthful. For example, on most diets you shed 75% fat and 25% muscle. On the EOD Diet, however, you lose about 99% fat and 1% muscle. And if you exercise while on the EOD Diet, you *gain* muscle. That's remarkable. And it's not the only remarkable "reset" produced by every-other-day dieting.

Not only does the EOD Diet lower LDL cholesterol, it specifically lowers the levels of the hard, dense LDL particles that do the most damage to your arteries. And people on the EOD Diet have an unusually large spike in levels of adiponectin, a hormone that protects your heart. Plus, a growing body of cellular animal and human research shows that every-other-day eating strengthens brain cells. I suspect those remarkable changes extend to appetite.

Every other day, you're allowed to eat all you want. But because you're on the EOD Diet, your body has a better idea: it decides to regulate appetite, so you don't overeat and hurt your health.

Stomach-shrinking. The very low-calorie intake of Diet Day may gradually shrink the stomach, cutting appetite.

No-binge psychology. The fact that you *can* binge on the Feast Day may *prevent* a binge. When foods are forbidden, you crave them and end up bingeing sooner or later. On the other hand, when foods are allowed, they're not as tempting and you can take them or leave them.

Tuning in to true hunger. You don't eat until lunch on Diet Day, so you experience *real hunger.* And that's a new experience for the average American, who eats so constantly during the day that he or she almost never experiences the body's *natural hunger cues*—the body letting the brain know when it's time to eat. Instead, most people experience only *emotional hunger cues*—the stress, anger, depression, anxiety, and boredom that drive us to eat for emotional comfort rather than physical well-being. On Diet Day, you learn what hunger feels like—and that newfound understanding extends to Feast Day.

Of course, you don't have to understand *why* the EOD Diet works in order to control your appetite; the EOD Diet controls appetite automatically!

ALLISON'S STORY: "THIS CAN'T BE A DIET!"

Weight loss: 7 pounds

Allison P. Davis, an editor at *Elle* magazine, wrote about the Every-Other-Day Diet in the February 2013 issue, in an article entitled "Halftime Diet." In the article, she used the terms I use in my scientific papers: *alternate-day fasting* for the EOD Diet; *fast day* for Diet Day; and *feed day* for Feast Day.

Allison had tried Weight Watchers and other diets. But, she wrote, "any decision I make to cut back instantly

(continued)

activates my instinct to gorge." What would happen to that "instinct" on the EOD Diet?

On Diet Days, she wrote, "it was a comfort just to know that at the stroke of midnight I could have whatever I wanted again. And it was freeing to stop counting calories and making trade-offs. I wasn't swapping points or keeping a diary; I was simply eating."

But after a Feast Day "involving mimosas, a fried chicken sandwich, and a side of bacon," she phoned Monica Klempel, PhD, a nutritionist who has helped me conduct many of the studies.

"This can't be a diet!" she shouted over the phone.

"Well, it sounds like you're doing it right," Dr. Klempel replied.

Allison wrote: "Fasting, Dr. Klempel explained, plays a mind game of sorts: Most subjects in both of Varady's studies tended to think they were consuming more calories on feed days than they really were. Though that fried chicken seemed unforgivably decadent, I'd eaten only half of it. This was occurring on most feed days: Once I got past the initial cravings, the natural desire for fruits and vegetables took over. At the office cafeteria, I'd steer toward the sushi bar rather than the grill. And the scale crept down: I lost a pound and a half the first week; seven by the end of the month."

After talking with Dr. Klempel, Allison talked to a dietitian who was skeptical that the EOD Diet would work long-term. Later, she called me and described the dietitian's doubts. People can and do stay on the diet long-term, I told her—

and the high-fat version of the EOD Diet makes it even more feasible.

She ended her article with this quote from me, and I'd say the same thing today: "It's really only having to diet half the time. People can really stick to that."

REMEMBER: HIGH-FAT IS ON THE FEAST DAY MENU

When I say you can eat *any* type of food you want on Feast Day, I mean *any* type of food—and that includes the high-fat foods found in the typical American diet. As I discussed in chapters 1 and 2, my studies show that dieters lose *more* weight when they eat high-fat foods on Diet Day and Feast Day. Yes, *more weight.*

For me, these studies confirm the essential principle and practice of the Every-Other-Day Diet: **You don't change *what* you're eating. You change your *pattern* of eating.** You consume 500 calories on Diet Day—eating any type of food. There is no calorie restriction on Feast Day—and you eat any type of food. *And that's it!* The EOD Diet is *simple.* The EOD Diet is *powerful.* Most importantly, the EOD Diet is *effective.*

ENJOY FEAST DAY!

I'd like to end this chapter with a brief pep talk about Feast Day—or maybe it's a pepperoni talk! Because on Feast Day you should have that pepperoni, and the pizza, and whatever other toppings, side dishes, beverages, and snacks strike your fancy. Truly, on Feast Day there are no restrictions and no forbidden foods. There are no rules whatsoever, unless "Enjoy yourself" is a rule!

Remember, the Every-Other-Day Diet works *because* you diet only every other day. The unrestricted day off from dieting gives your body the calories and nutrients it needs for a day of modified fasting. The modified fast creates a condition that helps you not overeat. Both days are necessary. Diet Day and Feast Day work *together* to produce sustained and safer weight loss.

If you're reading this book, it's likely that all the diets you've tried have failed. The Every-Other-Day Diet is unique—and uniquely effective. And Feast Day is the day of food and fun that makes it work!

EOD—EASY AS 1-2-3!

1. On Feast Day, eat all the food you want, and eat any kind of food you want.
2. Don't worry about bingeing on Feast Day—you won't.
3. You're not changing *what* you eat—you're changing your *pattern* of eating.

CHAPTER 4

Diet Day Recipes—Quick, Easy, and Delicious

These lunch and dinner recipes are only 400 calories, but they taste like a million!

In chapter 5, I present what is probably the simplest and easiest way to control calories on Diet Day: Eat store-bought frozen meals for lunch or dinner.

But maybe you'd rather prepare your own lunch or dinner on Diet Day. And if that's the case—if you're a person who enjoys perusing and choosing recipes, and making meals—you probably look for a couple of standard features in the recipes that you make on a regular basis. You want those recipes to be:

- *simple*, with a limited number of easy-to-find ingredients. Complex recipes are annoying.
- *speedy*, so you can make the recipe fast. You don't want to spend too much time in the kitchen. And if you're hungry, you want to eat *soon*.
- *scrumptious*, so the dish tastes good. Why bother making food if it's not tasty?
- *surprising*, so the meal is fun to eat, rather than the same-old, same-old. Variety is the spice of life (and of lunch and dinner).
- *satisfying*, with a meal that fills you up rather than leaves you hungry.

Well, you're in luck, because those benefits are just what the recipes in the Every-Other-Day Diet deliver. That's because our recipe developer, Stephanie Karpinske, MS, RD, is an old hand at developing delicious recipes for diets and diet books, and her weight-loss recipes appear regularly in national magazines like *Better Homes and Gardens* and *Family Circle*. For the recipes in the Every-Other-Day Diet, she made sure that all of the above criteria were met. She also made sure that:

- No recipe has an ingredient list of more than seven items. Simple as can be!
- Cooking and preparation times are always under 30 minutes, and frequently under 20 minutes. You're out of the kitchen fast!

Bill and I and our respective spouses tested all of the recipes, and we're pretty sure you'll agree with us that they are fast, easy, tasty, and fun. It's amazing how much freshness and originality Stephanie packed into these meals and snacks. And because the recipes feature appetite-satisfying protein and fiber, they're filling, too.

We've provided 28 days of 400-calorie lunches, 28 days of 400-calorie dinners, and 28 days of 100-calorie snacks. As you learned in chapter 2, you'll eat *either* lunch *or* dinner on Diet Day—your choice. Add the snack when it feels best to you, perhaps at midmorning, midafternoon, or at bedtime. We didn't create a meal plan out of these lunches, dinners, and snacks. That's because we wanted to give you maximum flexibility in choosing what meal to eat on Diet Day. Maybe you want to eat lunch on Monday, dinner on Wednesday, dinner on Friday, and lunch on Sunday. Go right ahead! Plus, feel free to mix and match the 28 snacks with any entrée. You can make *all* of them over two months of Diet Days. Or you can choose a few you especially like and make them over and over again. In other words, you won't need an executive assistant to follow the Every-Other-Day Diet.

And you won't need an executive chef either! When we reviewed the introductions to the recipe sections of many other diet books, we were struck by how complicated they were. There are endless lists of foods to eat and not to eat. There are "steps" and "phases" and "waves," time periods when you're asked to switch from one set of foods and one set of recipes to another. And the recipes themselves often seem like they would challenge even the most experienced chef, with long lists of ingredients and lengthy preparation times. No wonder most people don't stick with their diets!

You'll find none of those difficulties in the following recipes.

What you will find is easy preparation, good taste, and one simple dietary rule: stick to 500 calories on Diet Day.

A NOTE ABOUT BRANDS

When a brand-based product is mentioned (such as Thomas' Light Multi-Grain English Muffins, or Wild Garden Fire Roasted Red Pepper Hummus), it's best to use that exact product. Stephanie chose it either because it works best with the recipe or because the calorie count of that product is significantly lower than other similar products.

If you decide to use a different product, check the calorie count of the product in the recipe and the calorie count of the product you're substituting and make sure your substitution has the same amount of calories.

Sometimes when we list a product in a recipe, we say "such as..." (for example, "low-fat light sesame ginger dressing, such as Newman's Own Lite"). In that case, several brands are at the same level of calories (within 10 to 20 calories), but this product choice was the specific brand Stephanie used to make and test the recipe. This is particularly true of salad dressings. When you read "such as," it's fine to pick an alternate brand.

TIPS ON PREPARATION, SHOPPING, AND HEALTH

At the end of many of the recipes you'll find either a tip to ease shopping or preparation, or a Health Tip about a particular good-for-you ingredient. You should try to stick as closely as possible to the preparation guidelines we've suggested so as to ensure the right calorie count. For example, if using regular cheese didn't exceed the calorie count, we used regular cheese, rather than reduced-fat cheese, because my research shows that people who eat high-fat foods actually lose more weight on the EOD Diet, as long as they don't eat too many calories. However, sometimes regular cheese would exceed the calorie count, so the recipe includes the reduced-fat variety. When it comes to seasoning, though, feel free to add salt and pepper and other spices as you wish. Where salt is listed as an ingredient, we found the recipe tasted better with a dash of it; otherwise, follow your own preferences and enjoy!

400-CALORIE LUNCHES

Italian Quinoa Salad

¼ cup dry quinoa
2 ounces drained chunk light tuna in water
½ cup rinsed and drained canned garbanzo beans
½ small cucumber, peeled and chopped
5 kalamata olives, pitted and chopped
2 tablespoons light Italian dressing, such as Wish-Bone Light Italian

Cook quinoa according to package directions. Let cool. Place cooked quinoa in a medium bowl. Add remaining ingredients and mix to combine. If desired, chill before serving.

Health Tip: Quinoa (pronounced *keen-wah*) is a gluten-free grain: it doesn't have any of the gluten proteins found in wheat and rye that many folks are trying to avoid for better health. Quinoa has a mild flavor that mixes well with other ingredients, and it's rich in protein, making it a great choice for vegetarians.

Turkey and Avocado Sandwich

1 Arnold Sandwich Thins Roll
1 Laughing Cow Light Queso Fresco & Chipotle cheese wedge
4 ounces thinly sliced deli turkey breast
2–3 tomato slices
⅕ pitted and peeled avocado, thinly sliced

Split sandwich thin open. Spread one half of the thin with the cheese. Top with turkey, tomato, avocado, and remaining half of the sandwich thin.

Serve with 1 piece of fresh fruit or 1 single-serve package of any flavor Popchips.

Health Tip: Tomatoes are rich in lycopene, an anticancer compound. Eating avocado *with* tomatoes increases the body's absorption of lycopene by an amazing 200% to 400%.[1]

BBQ Chicken and Broccoli Wrap

3 ounces rotisserie chicken breast, shredded
⅓ cup drained canned corn
½ cup broccoli slaw
2 teaspoons jarred barbecue sauce
1 tablespoon reduced-fat ranch dressing
1 multigrain Flatout Soft 100% Whole Wheat Flatbread

Place chicken, corn, broccoli slaw, barbecue sauce, and ranch dressing in a medium bowl. Mix until everything is coated. Place mixture on the Flatout wrap and carefully roll up. If desired, cut in half before serving.

Preparation Tips: You can find broccoli slaw in the produce section, next to the bagged lettuce. For this recipe, you can also use plain cooked chicken breast. It has fewer calories than rotisserie chicken, but less flavor.

Tortellini Salad

1½ cups cooked Buitoni Light Four Cheese Ravioli*
1 cup fresh snow peas
½ cup chopped yellow sweet pepper
½ cup chopped red sweet pepper
2 tablespoons low-fat light sesame ginger dressing, such as
  Newman's Own Lite

Drain and cool ravioli, then add snow peas, sweet peppers, and dressing. If desired, chill before serving.

*Prepared according to package directions.

Shopping Tips: You'll find the Buitoni Light Four Cheese Ravioli in the refrigerator case. Also, snow peas and sugar snap peas are often confused, so make sure you buy the right ones! Snow peas are flat with a thin pod; sugar snap peas are plump with a thicker pod.

Black Bean and Corn Salad

¾ cup rinsed and drained canned black beans
⅔ cup drained canned corn
1 cup chopped green sweet pepper
1 small tomato, chopped
½ small peeled and pitted avocado, chopped
1 tablespoon red wine vinegar
¼ teaspoon ground cumin

Mix together all ingredients in a medium bowl. If desired, season with salt.

Health Tip: Several studies from Arizona State University show that adding vinegar to a meal helps control postmeal spikes of blood sugar, probably because the acetic acid in the vinegar blocks an enzyme that breaks down carbohydrates.[2]

Ham, Apple, and Cheddar Sandwich

2 teaspoons apple butter

1 Thomas' Light Multi-Grain English Muffin, toasted

4 ounces thinly sliced lean (96% fat-free) deli ham

1 small apple

1 (1-ounce) slice reduced-fat sharp cheddar cheese

Spread apple butter on bottom half of English muffin. Top with ham. Cut 3 to 4 thin slices from the apple and place on top of the ham. Cover ham with the cheddar cheese and muffin top. Slice the remaining apple and serve with the sandwich.

Health Tip: Reduced-fat cheese *isn't* reduced in calcium, a mineral many studies link to improved weight control.

Roast Beef Sub

⅓ cup drained and chopped jarred roasted red peppers

5 small kalamata olives, pitted and chopped

1 teaspoon red wine vinegar

1 whole-grain hot dog bun

4 ounces thinly sliced lean (96% fat-free) deli roast beef

1 (1-ounce) slice provolone cheese

Preheat oven to 350°F. Place red peppers, olives, and vinegar in a small bowl. Mix to combine, then set aside. Place hot dog bun on an oven-safe tray. Split bun open and top with roast beef and cheese. Bake for 2 to 3 minutes, or until bun is toasted and cheese is melted. Remove from oven and top melted cheese with pepper-olive mixture.

Health Tip: Roast beef is rich in protein, a super-satisfying macronutrient that helps control hunger.

Sesame Ginger Chicken Slaw

3 cups coleslaw mix

4 ounces cooked chicken breast, chopped

1 cup fresh snow peas

3 tablespoons low-fat light sesame ginger dressing, such as
    Newman's Own Lite

10 dry-roasted cashews, chopped

Place everything except the cashews in a large bowl. Mix until coleslaw is evenly coated with dressing. Let rest 10 minutes to allow dressing to soak into the slaw. Toss in cashews immediately before serving.

Health Tip: A study from the University of Montreal shows that cashew extracts are antidiabetic, helping muscles use blood sugar.[3]

Taco Salad

3 cups bagged mixed salad greens

¼ cup shredded reduced-fat cheddar cheese

4 ounces cooked chicken breast, shredded or chopped

½ red sweet pepper, seeded and chopped

1 tablespoon light ranch dressing

2 tablespoons jarred salsa

10 bite-sized round tortilla chips, broken into pieces

Place salad greens, cheese, chicken, and sweet pepper in a medium bowl. In a separate smaller bowl, stir together ranch dressing and salsa. Pour dressing mix over salad and toss to coat. Top with broken tortilla chips.

Health Tip: A mix of salad greens delivers far more calcium, vitamin C, and vitamin A than the same amount of iceberg lettuce.

Turkey and Hummus Wrap

¼ cup Wild Garden Fire Roasted Red Pepper Hummus
1 La Tortilla Factory Smart & Delicious 100 Calorie Tortilla
4 ounces thinly sliced deli turkey breast
5–6 leaves fresh baby spinach
3–4 tomato slices

Spread hummus on tortilla. Top with turkey, spinach, and tomato. Roll up and cut in half.

Serve with 1 piece of fresh fruit or a 100-calorie pack of any flavor SunChips.

Shopping and Preparation Tip: The calories in hummus vary by brand: the hummus used in this recipe has 70 calories per ¼ cup, but most other brands have 70 calories per 2 tablespoons. If you use another brand, check the label for calories per serving and adjust the amount accordingly.

Mango Chicken Salad

4 ounces cooked chicken breast, chopped
2 tablespoons chopped celery
2 tablespoons chopped red onion
5 dry-roasted almonds, chopped
¼ cup nonfat Greek yogurt
1 tablespoon mango chutney
2 Wasa Multi Grain Crispbread

Place chicken, celery, red onion, and almonds in a medium bowl. In a separate smaller bowl, mix together yogurt and chutney. Pour over chicken mixture and mix until combined. If desired, season with salt. Serve the salad on or with crispbread.

Health Tip: Studies show that almonds aid in weight control and deliver several other health benefits, including lowering high blood sugar and LDL cholesterol.[4]

Tuna and White Bean Salad

1 ounce (about ⅓ cup) uncooked medium shell pasta

4 ounces chunk light tuna in water, drained

½ cup rinsed and drained canned navy beans

½ medium cucumber, peeled and chopped

¼ cup reduced-fat feta cheese

2 tablespoons light Italian dressing, such as Wish-Bone Light Italian

Cook pasta according to package directions. Drain and let cool. Place pasta in a medium bowl. Add tuna, beans, cucumber, feta cheese, and dressing. Toss to coat. If desired, chill before serving.

Preparation Tip: Light tuna has 15 fewer calories per serving than albacore tuna, but a fishier taste. If you prefer a milder fish flavor, use albacore; 3 ounces is equivalent in calories to 4 ounces of light tuna.

Turkey Couscous Salad

¼ cup dry whole wheat couscous

3 ounces cooked turkey breast, cubed

1 small orange, peeled, sectioned, and cut into bite-sized pieces

1 tablespoon dried cranberries

1 green onion, chopped

2 tablespoons light cranberry walnut dressing, such as Newman's Own Lite

Cook couscous according to package directions. Let cool. Place couscous in a medium bowl. Add turkey, orange pieces, cranberries, green onion, and dressing. Toss to coat. If desired, chill before serving.

Preparation Tip: When making couscous, be sure to follow the cooking directions on the package closely. If you add too much water, you'll end up with soggy rather than fluffy grain. And if you cook the couscous too long, it can stick to the bottom of the pan.

Turkey and Pepperjack Bagel

1 Thomas' 100% Whole Wheat Bagel Thins bagel
1 tablespoon cherry preserves
3 ounces thinly sliced smoked deli turkey breast
1 (1-ounce) slice pepperjack cheese
1 leaf romaine lettuce

Split open the bagel thin. Spread cherry preserves on the bottom half. Top with turkey, cheese, and lettuce. Cut in half to serve.

Ham and Pear Wrap

1 tablespoon reduced-fat cream cheese
1 teaspoon Dijon mustard
1 multigrain medium (8-inch) tortilla
4 ounces thinly sliced lean (96% fat-free) deli ham
1 thin slice red onion, separated into rings
1 medium pear

Mix cream cheese and mustard together and spread on the tortilla. Top with ham and red onion. Cut pear into thin slices. Place a third of the pear slices on top of the red onion. Roll up the tortilla, then cut in half. Serve with the remaining pear slices.

Health Tip: Onions are one of the richest sources of quercetin, a powerful antioxidant that studies link to lower blood pressure, lower LDL cholesterol, fewer symptoms during allergy season, and less fatigue during exercise.[5]

Chicken and Pasta Soup

4 ounces cooked chicken breast, chopped
½ cup frozen mixed vegetables
3 cups chicken broth
1½ ounces (¼ cup) dry ditalini pasta

Combine chicken, vegetables, and broth in a small saucepan. Bring to a boil. Add pasta, then simmer for 10 to 12 minutes, or until pasta and vegetables are tender.

Ham and Bean Soup

4 ounces lean cooked ham, chopped
¾ cup rinsed and drained canned navy beans
½ small zucchini, chopped
½ yellow sweet pepper, seeded and chopped
2½ cups chicken broth
⅛ teaspoon ground black pepper

Combine all ingredients in a small saucepan. Bring to a boil, then simmer for 12 to 15 minutes, or until vegetables are tender.

Shopping Tip: There's a lot of variation in sodium (salt) levels in store-bought chicken broth, ranging from 400 to 900 mg per cup. To further confuse the situation, brands labeled "low sodium" aren't always the lowest. Check the Nutrition Facts panel on the label to see how much sodium you're actually getting.

Turkey and Orzo Soup

4 ounces cooked turkey breast, chopped
1 cup chopped kale
1 cup chopped white button mushrooms
3 cups chicken broth
1½ ounces (3 tablespoons) dry orzo
1 tablespoon shredded Parmesan cheese

Combine turkey, kale, mushrooms, and broth in a small saucepan. Bring to a boil, then add orzo and simmer for 10 to 12 minutes, or until vegetables are desired tenderness and orzo is cooked. Top with Parmesan cheese before serving.

Health Tip: Kale boosts the body's level of *nitric oxide*, a molecule that relaxes arteries and helps control blood pressure.

Edamame Penne Salad

1 ounce (⅓ cup) dry penne pasta

½ cup frozen shelled edamame, defrosted

½ yellow sweet pepper, seeded and chopped

½ cup grape tomatoes, halved

2 tablespoons light balsamic vinaigrette, such as Newman's Own Lite

2 tablespoons reduced-fat feta cheese

Cook pasta according to package directions. Drain and let cool. Place pasta in a medium bowl. Add remaining ingredients and toss to coat. If desired, chill before serving.

Health Tip: Edamame (pronounced *ed-ah-ma-may*) are immature green soybeans, served in their pods, a standard appetizer in Japanese restaurants. You can find them in the frozen food section of most supermarkets. You also can find edamame already shelled. You're using the pealike, fresh beans *inside* the pods (the pods aren't eaten). *Bonus:* edamame are rich in phytoestrogens, a plant-based, weaker version of estrogen that may help ease the symptoms of menopause.

Asian Chicken Salad

4 ounces cooked chicken breast, chopped

⅓ cup drained pineapple tidbits

1 tablespoon chopped red sweet pepper

5 almonds, chopped

½ cup precooked brown rice, such as Uncle Ben's Ready Rice

2 cups mixed salad greens

2 tablespoons low-fat/light sesame ginger dressing, such as Newman's Own Lite

Place all ingredients in a medium bowl. Gently toss to combine. If desired, chill before serving.

Health Tip: Pineapple is rich in bromelain, an enzyme that aids digestion and lowers inflammation.

Ham and Rice Salad

½ cup frozen peas, defrosted
½ cup precooked brown rice, such as Uncle Ben's Ready Rice
3 ounces lean cooked ham, chopped
1 Roma tomato (Italian plum tomato), chopped
2 cups chopped romaine lettuce
2 tablespoons reduced-fat ranch salad dressing

Place all ingredients in a medium bowl. Gently toss to combine. If desired, chill before serving.

Health Tip: Brown rice is a whole grain. A study from Wake Forest University shows that eating 2 to 3 servings of whole grains daily can lower your risk of heart disease by 21%, compared to the risk of people who hardly eat any whole grains.[6]

Thai Noodle Salad

1 ounce dry whole wheat spaghetti
½ sweet red pepper, seeded and chopped
3 ounces cooked chicken breast, shredded or chopped
2 green onions, chopped
2 tablespoons bottled peanut sauce
10 dry-roasted peanuts, whole or chopped

Cook spaghetti according to package directions. Drain and let cool. Place spaghetti in a medium bowl. Add sweet pepper, chicken, green onion, peanut sauce, and peanuts. Gently toss to combine. If desired, chill before serving.

Health Tip: Peanuts get a bad rap for causing allergies, but if you're *not* allergic to them, they're very good for you. Research shows roasted peanuts eaten with a meal can help control blood sugar.[7]

Chicken and Bacon Lettuce Wraps

3 slices ready-to-serve fully cooked bacon
4 ounces cooked chicken breast, shredded or chopped
½ cup diced fresh tomato
2 tablespoons reduced-fat ranch dressing
2–3 large leaves butterhead (Bibb) lettuce

Heat bacon according to package directions. Cool, then crumble. Place bacon, chicken, tomato, and dressing in a medium bowl. Mix to combine. Fill lettuce leaves with chicken mixture, then roll leaves up to serve.

Serve with 1 small piece of fruit.

Corn and Bean Burrito

⅔ cup fat-free refried beans
2 tablespoons jarred salsa
1 multigrain medium (8-inch) tortilla
¼ cup drained canned corn
⅓ cup shredded lettuce
¼ cup reduced-fat shredded Mexican taco cheese blend

Place beans in a covered microwave-safe dish and heat on high for 45 seconds to 1 minute, stirring halfway through. If beans aren't heated through, microwave a few seconds more. Remove from microwave and stir in salsa. Spread bean mixture on the tortilla. Top with corn, lettuce, and cheese. Roll ends of tortilla toward the center, then roll up from the side to serve.

Loaded Baked Potato

1 medium russet potato
2 tablespoons light vegetable dip or French onion dip
¼ teaspoon ground black pepper
1 cup chopped frozen broccoli
3 ounces lean cooked ham, chopped

Scrub potato and prick sides several times with a fork. Place in microwave and cook on high for 5 to 6 minutes or until potato is tender. Split open the top of the potato and scoop out two-thirds of the flesh into a small bowl. Add dip and pepper, then mix to combine. Scoop potato mixture back into potato. Cook broccoli according to package directions. If desired, warm ham in the microwave. Top potato with broccoli and ham.

Health Tip: Potatoes are loaded with potassium, an important mineral for preventing and lowering high blood pressure.

Spicy Beef Chili

4 ounces 95% lean ground beef
1 cup canned diced tomatoes, undrained
⅔ cup rinsed and drained canned pinto beans
½ cup jarred salsa
½ cup water
½ teaspoon chili seasoning or chili powder
1 tablespoon reduced-fat cheddar cheese

Brown ground beef in a small to medium saucepan over medium-high heat until cooked through. Drain fat, if necessary. Add diced tomatoes, beans, salsa, water, and chili seasoning. Bring to a boil, then simmer for 10 to 15 minutes. Top with cheese before serving.

Health Tip: Pinto beans deliver *soluble fiber*, which can help banish belly fat.

Roast Beef with Cucumber Sauce

½ cucumber, peeled, seeded, and chopped
¼ cup reduced-fat sour cream
1 tablespoon chopped red onion
½ tablespoon chopped fresh dill
⅛ teaspoon salt
1 large (6½-inch diameter) whole wheat pita bread
4 ounces thinly sliced deli roast beef

Place cucumber, sour cream, onion, dill, and salt in a small bowl. Mix well to make sauce. Cut pita in half and open. Divide roast beef among pita halves. Top with cucumber sauce.

Health Tip: A study in *Stroke* links eating cucumbers (and other fruits and vegetables with white flesh, like apples and pears) to a 52% lower risk of stroke.[8]

Mediterranean Tuna-Topped Tomato

5 ounces chunk light tuna in water, drained
½ tablespoon olive oil
5 small kalamata olives, pitted and chopped
1 tablespoon chopped red onion
¼ cup reduced-fat feta cheese
1 medium tomato

Place tuna, oil, olives, red onion, and feta cheese in a small bowl. Gently mix to combine. Cut out tomato stem; then slice tomato into quarters. Top with tuna mixture.

Health Tip: Feta cheese is rich in *conjugated linoleic acid*, a type of fat that can help control weight, cool inflammation, strengthen immunity, and fight cancer.

400-CALORIE DINNERS

Cornmeal-Crusted Cod

1 (4-ounce) piece cod, hake, haddock, or tilapia, about ½ inch
    thick
¼ cup low-fat buttermilk
2 tablespoons cornmeal
½ teaspoon lemon-pepper seasoning
⅛ teaspoon dried dill or parsley

Preheat oven to 425°F. Place cod in a ziptop plastic bag. Pour
buttermilk into the bag and seal. Turn the bag side to side to coat the
cod. Set aside. Combine cornmeal, lemon-pepper seasoning, and dill
in a small bowl. Remove cod from bag and place it in the cornmeal
mixture. Turn to coat all sides of the cod. Place cod in a shallow
baking pan that has been lightly coated with nonstick cooking spray.
Lightly spray the top of the fish with the cooking spray. Bake for 12 to
15 minutes, turning once. Fish is done when it flakes easily with a fork.

Serve with ¾ cup Ore-Ida Steam n' Mash Cut Red Potatoes,
prepared according to package directions.

Health Tip: Even a little bit of parsley does the body good. Research
shows the herb may fight heart disease, diabetes, and cancer.

Spaghetti and Meatballs

1½ ounces dry multigrain spaghetti, such as Barilla Plus
7 frozen meatless meatballs, such as MorningStar Farms Meal
    Starters Veggie Meatballs; or 4 frozen Italian-style turkey
    meatballs
½ cup marinara sauce
½ teaspoon Italian seasoning; or ¼ teaspoon each dried basil
    and dried oregano
⅛ teaspoon crushed red pepper (optional)

Cook pasta according to package directions. Drain and set aside. Heat meatballs according to package directions. Put marinara sauce and seasonings (and red pepper, if desired) in a small saucepan and simmer until sauce is warmed. Add meatballs to sauce and stir to combine. Serve meatballs and sauce over cooked spaghetti.

Serve with ½ cup cooked green beans.

Health Tip: Oregano is another health-giving spice; research links it to the prevention of a wide range of diseases and conditions, including infections, prediabetes, and high cholesterol.

Pepperoni Pizza

1 Flatout Light Italian Herb Flatbread
¼ cup drained canned crushed tomatoes with Italian herbs
10 small slices pepperoni
4 white button mushrooms, sliced thin
⅓ cup Italian five-cheese-blend shredded cheese
Chopped fresh basil

Preheat oven to 425°F. Place flatbread on a baking sheet. Top with crushed tomatoes, spreading evenly to cover. Add pepperoni slices, mushrooms, and cheese. Bake for 5 to 7 minutes, or until cheese melts and starts to turn golden brown. Remove from oven and top with chopped basil.

Serve with tossed salad made using 2 cups bagged mixed salad greens, ½ cup grape tomatoes, and 2 tablespoons light Italian dressing.

Shopping Tip: The Flatout company makes flatbreads in different shapes, sizes, and flavors, which you can find in the bread aisle or produce section of most grocery stores.

Chicken Enchiladas

2 ounces rotisserie chicken breast, shredded

½ cup rinsed and drained canned black beans

¼ cup jarred enchilada sauce, *divided*

2 tablespoons reduced-fat cheddar cheese, *divided*

2 small (6-inch) corn tortillas; or 1 medium (8-inch) multigrain
tortilla

Preheat oven to 400°F. Combine chicken, beans,
2 tablespoons of the enchilada sauce, and *1 tablespoon* of the
cheese in a medium bowl. Place mixture on the tortillas. Carefully
roll up tortillas and place in a small baking dish. (It's okay if filling
spills out of the sides.) Spoon remaining enchilada sauce over top
of the enchiladas, then top with remaining cheese. Bake for 10 to
12 minutes, or until filling is warmed.

Preparation Tip: You could also use plain cooked chicken breast. It has
fewer calories than rotisserie chicken, but also has less flavor.

BBQ Pork Chops with Apple-Topped Sweet Potato

½ teaspoon barbecue seasoning blend

1 (4-ounce) lean boneless pork chop, about ½ inch thick

1 medium (5-ounce) sweet potato

½ cup applesauce

¼ teaspoon cinnamon

Rub barbecue seasoning on both sides of the pork chop. Spray a
medium skillet with nonstick cooking spray. Place pork chop in skillet
and cook over medium-high heat for 4 to 5 minutes per side, or until
pork is cooked through (internal temperature of at least 145°F). As
the pork chop cooks, scrub the sweet potato, then prick all around
the outside of it with a fork. Microwave on high for 7 to 10 minutes,
or until tender. Split top of the potato open. Mix applesauce with
cinnamon. Top sweet potato with applesauce. Serve with pork chop.

Health Tip: Sweet potatoes are loaded with the antioxidant *alpha-carotene*. A 10-year study from the Centers for Disease Control and Prevention showed that people with the highest blood levels of alpha-carotene had a 39% lower risk of death during the study than people with low levels.[9]

Steak and Peppers

1 (4-ounce) sirloin steak, about ¾ inch thick
2 cloves garlic, *divided*
Salt and ground black pepper
½ tablespoon olive oil
½ green sweet pepper, seeded and cut into thin slices
½ red sweet pepper, seeded and cut into thin slices
⅓ small onion, cut into thin slices

Preheat broiler. Trim steak of any visible fat, then place on tray of broiler pan. Cut *1 clove* of garlic in half and rub the cut sides on both sides of the steak. Sprinkle with salt and black pepper. Broil 4 inches from heat, turning once, for 8 to 12 minutes, or until beef reaches desired doneness (145°F for medium rare, 160°F for medium, and 170°F for well done). Keep an eye on the steak while it broils, as it can burn quickly.

For pepper mixture, heat oil in a medium skillet. Add sweet peppers and onion. Sauté for a few minutes over medium-high heat. If peppers start to burn, add water, a tablespoon at a time, as needed. Chop the remaining clove of garlic and add to the skillet. Continue sautéing a few minutes more, until peppers and onions are just tender. Serve peppers and onions with the steak.

Preparation Tip: When you're cooking with very little or no fat, food sometimes sticks to the pan. If that happens, add a small amount of water to the pan, 1 tablespoon at a time. Be careful: water can splatter when you add it to a hot skillet.

Cheesy Burger

5 ounces 95% lean ground beef
¼ cup shredded sharp cheddar cheese
1 tablespoon finely chopped onion
⅛ teaspoon salt
⅛ teaspoon ground black pepper
1 Sara Lee Delightful Wheat Hamburger Bun
Optional toppers: lettuce, tomato, ketchup, mustard, pickles

Preheat broiler. Place beef, cheese, onion, salt, and pepper in a small to medium bowl. Mix together and form into a patty. Put burger on rack of a broiler pan. Broil 4 inches from the heat for 10 to 13 minutes or until desired doneness (145°F for medium rare, 160°F for medium, and 170°F for well done). Remove burger from broiler and serve on the bun with any of the optional toppers.

Health Tip: Surprise! Black pepper is a health food. It's rich in *piperine*, which research shows may help ease arthritis, lower blood pressure, prevent heart disease, and prevent Alzheimer's.[10]

Chicken Parmesan

1 (4-ounce) skinless, boneless chicken breast
2 teaspoons olive oil
2 tablespoons Italian-style panko bread crumbs
1 tablespoon grated Parmesan cheese
¼ cup jarred marinara sauce
¼ cup shredded mozzarella cheese

Preheat oven to 425°F. Place chicken on a baking sheet. Rub oil on both sides of the chicken. In a small shallow bowl, mix together bread crumbs and Parmesan cheese. Place chicken in the bread crumb mixture and turn to coat, pressing bread crumbs to chicken so they stick. Place chicken back on baking sheet. Bake for 20 to 25 minutes, or until chicken is cooked through (internal temperature of 170°F), turning once. Remove from oven and top with marinara sauce and mozzarella cheese. Return chicken to oven and bake a few minutes more until cheese is melted.

Shopping Tip: Store-bought marinara sauce is often high in sugar; some brands contain as much as 10 grams per serving. Check labels and choose the brand with the lowest amount of sugar. Or look for a variety that says "no sugar added."

BBQ Salmon with Mango Salsa

1 (4-ounce) fresh wild Atlantic skinless salmon filet, about
      ½ inch thick
2 tablespoons jarred barbecue sauce

For salsa:

1 cup chopped fresh mango
2 tablespoons chopped red onion
½ small cucumber, peeled and chopped
1 tablespoon chopped fresh cilantro
Juice from ½ small lime

Preheat broiler. Place salmon on tray of a broiler pan. Broil 4 inches from heat for 4 minutes. Remove from oven and brush with barbecue sauce. Broil for 2 minutes. Remove from oven again, flip the salmon, and brush the other side with the sauce. Broil for another 2 minutes, or until fish flakes easily with a fork. For salsa, place mango, onion, cucumber, cilantro, and lime juice in a small to medium bowl. Mix to combine, and serve with the salmon.

Health Tip: Oily salmon is loaded with omega-3 fat, a fat that is good for nearly every part of your body, including your brain (where it brightens mood), arteries (keeping them flexible and free of plaque), joints (easing aches and pains), and eyes (helping prevent cataracts and other age-related eye problems).[11]

Chicken Stir-Fry

4 ounces raw chicken breast tenderloins, cut into ¾-inch-thick strips

1½ cups frozen stir-fry vegetables

2 tablespoons bottled stir-fry sauce

1 cup precooked brown rice, such as Uncle Ben's Ready Rice

Lightly coat a medium skillet with nonstick cooking spray. Add chicken tenders and stir-fry over medium-high heat for 4 to 5 minutes. Add frozen vegetables and stir-fry sauce. Cook for 3 to 4 minutes more, or until chicken is cooked through and vegetables reach desired doneness. Serve over brown rice.

Ravioli Vegetable Toss

½ medium yellow summer squash, chopped

1 cup cherry tomatoes, halved

⅓ cup chicken broth

2 cups fresh baby spinach

1 cup cooked Buitoni Light Four Cheese Ravioli*

3 tablespoons shredded Parmesan cheese

Spray a medium to large skillet with nonstick cooking spray. Add yellow squash and tomatoes and sauté over medium-high heat for 2 to 3 minutes. Add broth and spinach and continue to sauté for 4 to 5 minutes more, or until squash is tender. Stir in cooked ravioli just to combine. Remove from heat. Top with cheese before serving.

* Prepared according to package directions.

Shopping Tip: You'll find Buitoni Light Four Cheese Ravioli in the refrigerator case.

Fettuccine with Cream Sauce

1 ounce reduced-fat or "⅓ less fat" cream cheese
¼ cup skim milk
⅛ teaspoon salt
1 tablespoon grated Parmesan cheese
½ cup frozen peas, defrosted
1¼ cups Buitoni fettuccine*
Coarse-ground black pepper

Whisk together cream cheese, milk, and salt in a small saucepan to make sauce. Bring to a boil, stirring constantly. Stir in cheese; then simmer over medium heat until mixture starts to bubble and thicken, stirring occasionally. Stir in peas. Pour sauce over prepared fettuccine and toss until sauce coats the pasta. Season with pepper.

* Prepared according to package directions.

Shopping Tip: You'll find Buitoni fettuccine in the refrigerator case.

Mini Meat Loaf with Mashed Potatoes

5 ounces 95% lean ground beef
1 teaspoon bread crumbs
1 teaspoon dry onion soup mix
2 teaspoons ketchup

Preheat oven to 450°F. Place beef, bread crumbs, soup mix, and ketchup in a small to medium bowl. Mix well to combine. Form mixture into a small oval-shaped loaf and place on rack of a broiler pan. Bake for 15 to 20 minutes, or until cooked through (internal temperature of at least 160°F). Keep an eye on the meat loaf as it cooks, as it can easily burn at this temperature.

Serve with 1¼ cups Ore-Ida Steam n' Mash Garlic Seasoned Potatoes, prepared according to package directions.

Chicken Nachos

20 mini round tortilla chips
2 ounces cooked chicken, shredded or chopped
½ cup rinsed and drained canned black beans
½ cup reduced-fat Mexican-blend cheese
1 Roma tomato (Italian plum tomato), diced; or 2 tablespoons
    jarred salsa
5 jarred, sliced jalapeños (optional)

Preheat oven to 375°F. Spread tortilla chips out on a baking tray so that they're touching but not piled on top of each other. Evenly top chips with chicken, beans, and cheese. Bake for 5 to 8 minutes, or until cheese is melted. Remove from oven and top with diced tomato and, if desired, jalapeños.

Health Tip: The jalapeños in the recipe might help you shed pounds. They're rich in *capsaicin*, a compound that many studies show helps control appetite.[12]

Sautéed Shrimp with Kale and Pine Nuts

2 teaspoons olive oil
4 ounces peeled and deveined shrimp, tails removed
1 clove garlic, sliced thin
1 cup chopped kale
½ cup rinsed and drained canned navy beans
1 tablespoon pine nuts

Heat oil in a medium skillet. Add shrimp and sauté over medium-high heat for 2 to 3 minutes. Add garlic and kale. Saute for 4 to 5 minutes more, or until shrimp are opaque. Stir in beans. Remove from heat. Sprinkle with pine nuts before serving.

Chicken with Spinach and Tomatoes

1 (5-ounce) boneless, skinless chicken breast
1 tablespoon olive oil
3 cups fresh baby spinach
1 clove garlic, sliced thin
¾ cup grape tomatoes
⅓ cup chicken broth
6 kalamata olives, pitted and sliced

Cut chicken into ¾-inch-wide strips. Heat oil in a medium to large skillet. Add chicken and sauté over medium-high heat for 3 to 4 minutes. Add spinach, garlic, and tomatoes. Sauté for 2 to 3 minutes more. Add broth and olives. Let simmer for 5 to 8 minutes, stirring occasionally, until chicken is cooked through and tomatoes are tender.

Health Tip: Garlic is great for you. Decades of scientific studies on garlic and health show that regular intake may help prevent many age-related diseases, including heart disease, stroke, cancer, dementia, arthritis, and cataracts.

Scallops with Pineapple Salsa

5 ounces fresh or frozen scallops
½ teaspoon Cajun seasoning
2 teaspoons olive oil

For salsa:

1½ cups fresh chopped pineapple
2 tablespoons chopped red onion
½ small jalapeño pepper, seeded and chopped
7 almonds, coarsely chopped

Thaw scallops, if frozen. Rinse and pat dry with a paper towel. Place in a medium bowl with the Cajun seasoning and toss until lightly coated. Heat oil in a medium skillet. Add scallops and cook over medium-high heat for 4 to 5 minutes, or until scallops are opaque throughout. Remove from heat. For salsa, place pineapple, red onion, jalapeños, and almonds in a medium bowl and toss to combine. Serve salsa with scallops.

Health Tip: Enjoy that olive oil! A Spanish study on the Mediterranean Diet, published in the *New England Journal of Medicine*, shows that the diet can reduce heart attacks and strokes by 30%, compared to a low-fat diet, and that olive oil is probably the diet's most heart-healthy ingredient.

Penne Primavera

⅔ cup (2 ounces) dry penne
1 tablespoon olive oil
½ small zucchini, cut into thin strips
1 yellow or orange sweet pepper, seeded and cut into thin strips
1 cup sliced portobello or white button mushrooms
⅓ cup chicken broth

Cook pasta according to package directions. Drain and set aside. Heat oil in a medium to large skillet. Add zucchini, sweet pepper, and mushrooms and sauté over medium-high heat for 5 to 6 minutes. Add broth and continue sautéing a few minutes more, until vegetables are tender. Stir in the cooked pasta before serving.

Shopping Tip: When buying pasta, try one of the many whole-grain blends now available. They have more nutrients and fiber than white pasta, yet taste almost the same.

Egg and Cheese Casserole

2 large eggs
½ cup low-fat milk
¼ teaspoon grainy mustard

¼ teaspoon ground black pepper
1 slice whole wheat bread, torn into bite-sized pieces
1 slice ready-to-serve fully cooked bacon, chopped
¼ cup shredded cheddar cheese, *divided*

Preheat oven to 400°F. Crack eggs into a small bowl. Add
milk, mustard, and pepper. Whisk until combined. Set aside.
In an individual-sized casserole dish, place bread, bacon, and
3 *tablespoons* of the cheese. Toss lightly to combine. Pour egg
mixture on top. Bake for 20 minutes, then remove from oven and top
with remaining *1 tablespoon* cheese. Return to oven and bake for 5 to
10 minutes more, or until knife inserted in center comes out clean.

Health Tip: We've included this breakfast-like recipe among the dinners
because some folks adore breakfast and miss not eating it on the EOD
Diet. Don't be afraid of eggs, bacon, and cheese on Diet Day. Studies
show that their hearty dose of fat and protein helps you feel full for
hours, reducing hunger.[13] And my research shows you can eat *anything*
on Diet Day and still improve risk factors for heart disease.

Sirloin Steak with Mushroom Sauce

¼ teaspoon ground black pepper
⅛ teaspoon garlic salt
1 (4-ounce) sirloin steak, about ¾ inch thick
1 green onion, chopped (optional)

For mushroom sauce:

1 cup sliced portobello mushrooms
1 cup sliced white button mushrooms
⅓ cup light Alfredo sauce, such as Ragú Light Parmesan
   Alfredo

Preheat broiler. Combine black pepper and garlic salt in a small
bowl. Rub over both sides of the steak. Place steak on rack of a broiler
pan and broil 3 inches from the heat, turning once, for 8 to 12 minutes,

or until steak reaches desired doneness (internal temperature 145°F for medium rare, 160°F for medium, and 170°F for well done). While steak cooks, prepare mushroom sauce. Spray a medium skillet with nonstick cooking spray. Add mushrooms and sauté over medium-high heat for 5 to 7 minutes, adding water, 1 tablespoon at a time, if needed, to keep mushrooms from burning. Stir in Alfredo sauce and cook for 3 to 4 minutes more, or until sauce is heated through. Pour sauce over steak. If desired, top with green onion.

Health Tip: White button mushrooms strengthen the immune system, report scientists at Tufts University in the *British Journal of Nutrition*.[14]

Chicken Cacciatore

⅓ cup (1½ ounces) dry rotini pasta
1 (4-ounce) boneless, skinless chicken breast
½ green sweet pepper, seeded and chopped
1 cup sliced white button mushrooms
1 cup canned diced tomatoes with garlic and basil, undrained

Cook pasta according to package directions. Drain and set aside. Cut chicken breast into bite-sized pieces. Spray a medium skillet with nonstick cooking spray. Add chicken and cook over medium-high heat for 2 to 3 minutes, just to brown the outside of the chicken. Add pepper and mushrooms and sauté for 4 to 5 minutes more, or until peppers are tender. Add diced tomatoes. Reduce heat and simmer about 5 minutes more. Stir in cooked pasta before serving.

BBQ Bacon and Pineapple Pizza

½ of a Boboli mini (8-inch) pizza crust
1 tablespoon jarred barbecue sauce
3 slices fully cooked Canadian bacon, such as Oscar Mayer

1 tablespoon chopped red onion

⅓ cup drained canned pineapple tidbits

¼ cup Italian five-cheese-blend shredded cheese

Preheat oven to 425°F. Place pizza crust half on a baking sheet. Spread barbecue sauce on top. Add Canadian bacon, red onion, and pineapple. Sprinkle cheese on top. Bake for 10 to 12 minutes, or until cheese is bubbly and lightly browned.

Rigatoni in Tomato Cream Sauce

¾ cup (2 ounces) dry rigatoni pasta

¾ cup jarred marinara sauce

⅓ cup 1% low-fat milk

¼–½ teaspoon red pepper flakes

2 tablespoons grated Parmesan cheese

Cook pasta according to package directions. Drain and set aside. Place marinara sauce, milk, and red pepper flakes in a small saucepan. Bring to a boil; then reduce heat and stir in cheese. Simmer uncovered for 10 to 12 minutes, or until sauce thickens, stirring occasionally. Stir in cooked pasta.

Chicken and Bean Quesadillas

2 small (fajita-size) flour tortillas

¼ cup canned fat-free refried beans

2 ounces cooked chicken breast, shredded or chopped

2 tablespoons reduced-fat shredded Mexican taco cheese blend

⅕ peeled and pitted avocado, mashed

Spray a medium skillet with nonstick cooking spray. Place 1 tortilla in the skillet. Spread refried beans on top. Top with chicken and cheese. Place the other tortilla on a plate. Spread one side with the mashed avocado. Place the tortilla, avocado side down, on top of the other tortilla. Press the top of the tortilla lightly so the quesadilla will hold together when you flip it. Spray the top with nonstick cooking spray. Cook quesadilla over medium to medium-high heat for 4 to 5 minutes per side, or until cheese is melted and tortillas are lightly browned.

> **Health Tip:** Avocados are the best source of *monounsaturated fats*, which studies show can help you control weight, lower LDL cholesterol, and balance blood sugar.

Pork Chop with Sautéed Apples and Onions

1 teaspoon olive oil
1 (5-ounce) lean boneless pork chop, about ½ inch thick
⅓ small sweet onion, sliced thin
1 small apple, cored and sliced thin
½ cup chicken broth
1 tablespoon balsamic vinegar

Heat oil in a medium to large skillet. Add pork chop and cook over medium-high heat for 4 to 5 minutes per side, or until cooked through (internal temperature of at least 145°F). Transfer chop to a plate and cover to keep warm. Place onion and apple in the skillet, sautéing for 1 to 2 minutes to lightly brown the outsides. Pour in broth and balsamic vinegar. Bring to a boil, then simmer for 8 to 10 minutes, or until onions and apples are tender. (If apple-and-onion mixture sticks to the pan, add a small amount of water.) Serve apple mixture with pork chop.

> **Health Tip:** An apple a day might keep the cardiologist away. Researchers from Ohio State University found that people eating an apple a day for just one month had a "tremendous" (40%) decrease in oxidized LDL cholesterol, the type of LDL that does the most damage to arteries.[15]

Steak Tacos

1 (4-ounce) sirloin steak
½ cup canned diced tomatoes with green chilies, such as
    Ro-Tel Tomatoes & Green Chilies, undrained
2 small corn taco shells, such as Old El Paso
½ cup shredded lettuce
2 tablespoons reduced-fat shredded cheddar cheese

Cut steak into thin strips. Spray a medium skillet with nonstick cooking spray. Place steak strips in skillet and sauté for 5 to 6 minutes over medium-high heat. Add diced tomatoes and cook for 5 to 6 minutes more, or until most of the liquid has evaporated. Divide beef-tomato mixture between the two taco shells. Top with shredded lettuce and cheese.

Chicken with Roasted Dijon Potatoes

1¼ cups diced red potatoes
2 teaspoons olive oil
1 teaspoon Dijon mustard
⅛ teaspoon salt
1 (5-ounce) chicken breast
2 tablespoons Lawry's Herb & Garlic Marinade with
    Lemon Juice

Preheat oven to 425°F. Place red potatoes, oil, mustard, and salt in a small bowl. Mix to coat, then transfer to a shallow oven-safe pan. Place chicken in a separate oven-safe baking dish, lined with foil. Pour marinade over the chicken, turning to coat. Place chicken and potatoes in oven. Bake for 20 to 25 minutes, or until potatoes are tender and chicken is cooked through (internal temperature of 170°F). If chicken is done before the potatoes, remove it from oven and cover to keep warm. Serve chicken with the potatoes.

Preparation Tip: The marinade contains sugar, and any remnants that run off the chicken tend to stick to the pan. Lining the baking pan with foil will make cleanup quick and easy.

Spicy Sausage and Rice

1 Al Fresco Spicy Jalapeño Chicken Sausage link
½ cup drained canned corn
½ cup rinsed and drained canned black beans
½ cup precooked brown rice, such as Uncle Ben's Ready Rice
2 tablespoons bottled salsa

Follow package instructions for preparing the sausage. Set aside. In a small microwave-safe bowl, combine corn, black beans, rice, and salsa. Microwave on high for 1 minute. Remove from microwave and stir. If needed, microwave another 30 seconds to 1 minute, or until mixture is warmed. Serve prepared sausage link with rice, corn, and bean mixture.

Shopping and Preparation Tips: You'll usually find Al Fresco Spicy Jalapeño Chicken Sausage links in the refrigerator case, near the prepacked deli meats. Rinsing canned beans removes a lot of the sodium, so before using, place the beans in a colander, rinse well with cold water, then let them sit for a minute to drain.

100-CALORIE SNACKS

Hummus-Cucumber Boats

1 medium cucumber
¼ cup Wild Garden Fire Roasted Red Pepper Hummus (or other desired flavor)
Paprika or salt to taste (optional)

Halve cucumber lengthwise. Use a spoon to hollow out the center of each cucumber half, removing the seeds. Spread

2 tablespoons hummus in each cucumber half. Sprinkle with paprika and/or salt, if desired.

Berry Smoothie Pops

⅓ cup plain nonfat Greek yogurt
¼ cup orange juice
¼ cup blueberries (fresh or frozen)
¼ cup strawberries (fresh or frozen)
Popsicle mold; or a 4- to 6-ounce plastic cup
Popsicle stick

Place yogurt, juice, and fruit in a blender or small food processor and blend or process until smooth. Pour mixture into a small (4- to 6-ounce) popsicle mold or plastic cup. Place popsicle stick upright in the middle of the popsicle mold section or cup and freeze until solid. Remove popsicle from mold or cup and serve.

Health Tip: Berries are superfruits. New studies show that regularly eating blueberries or strawberries can help strengthen the immune system, lower blood pressure, balance blood sugar, improve memory, and even help prevent precancerous lesions from turning into cancer.

Fruit with Cheese Spread

1 Laughing Cow Light Blue Cheese Wedge
½ small apple, cut into slices
½ small pear, cut into slices

Spread blue cheese onto apple and pear slices.

Peanut Butter and Banana Square

1 teaspoon creamy peanut butter
1 (2½-inch) graham cracker square
¼ of a small (6-inch) banana, cut into slices

Spread peanut butter onto graham cracker. Top with sliced bananas.

Health Tip: Worried that eating a banana might spike your blood sugar? Relax. A study in the *International Journal of Food Sciences and Nutrition* shows that a banana is a healthy snack for anybody trying to regulate glucose levels, including people with diabetes.[16]

Greek Yogurt Parfait

½ of a 6-ounce container of Chobani Greek nonfat vanilla
   yogurt
2 strawberries, hulled and sliced
¼ cup Berry Berry Kix cereal

Place yogurt in a parfait glass. Top with sliced berries and cereal.

Health Tip: Greek yogurt is regular yogurt that's been strained or filtered to remove the whey, giving it a creamier consistency and tangier taste; it has half the sugar and nearly double the protein of regular yogurt.

Jicama Sticks

2 (1-ounce) slices deli turkey
1 teaspoon Dijon mustard
¾ cup peeled, sliced jicama*

Place turkey slices on a plate. Spread with Dijon mustard. Cut turkey into enough strips to cover each jicama stick. Wrap the mustard side of the turkey around each jicama stick.
*Slice into thick matchsticks.

Health Tip: Jicama is a turniplike plant with a sweet/starchy flavor somewhat similar to an apple. It's rich in fiber and vitamin C.

Chocolate Stack

1 teaspoon creamy almond butter
1 Dove Rich Dark chocolate square
4 strawberries, hulled

Spread almond butter on chocolate square. Slice one of the strawberries and place slices on top of chocolate square. Serve with remaining whole strawberries.

Health Tip: Dark chocolate is loaded with antioxidants that protect your arteries. Research shows that regularly eating a small amount of dark chocolate can help lower blood pressure, LDL cholesterol, and the risk of heart disease and stroke. It can even help lower the risk of a *second* heart attack![17]

Trail Mix

½ cup Honey Kix cereal
¼ cup Cheerios cereal
15 raisins

Mix everything together in a small bowl.

Health Tip: A study from Canadian researchers shows that eating raisins as a snack can help you feel fuller and eat fewer calories afterward, compared to eating grapes, potato chips, or cookies.[18]

Garden Fresh Toast

½ of an Arnold Sandwich Thins Roll
2 tablespoons Wild Garden Sun Dried Tomato Hummus
½ small cucumber, sliced
Salt (optional)

Toast the sandwich thin. Spread the top with hummus; then top with sliced cucumbers. If desired, lightly sprinkle with salt.

Tomatoes, Peppers, and Cheese

½ medium tomato
½ yellow sweet pepper, seeded
1 (1-ounce) stick mozzarella string cheese

Coarsely chop tomato and sweet pepper and place in a small bowl. Cut string cheese into small pieces. Add cheese to the bowl with the tomato and peppers and toss to combine.

Mock Apple Crisp

½ cup unsweetened applesauce
⅛–¼ teaspoon cinnamon
¼ cup Cinnamon Toast Crunch cereal

Place applesauce in a microwave-safe bowl. Stir in cinnamon. Microwave on high for 20 to 30 seconds, or until applesauce is warmed. Place cereal in a separate bowl. Use the back of a spoon to lightly crush cereal. Top warmed applesauce with crushed cereal.

Health Tip: Cinnamon acts like glucose-controlling insulin in the body; studies show even a little bit of cinnamon with a meal can help balance postmeal blood sugar.[19]

Fruity Waffle Sticks

1 Eggo Nutri-Grain Low Fat Waffle, toasted
2 teaspoons reduced-fat cream cheese
1 teaspoon Polaner All Fruit Spreadable Fruit (any flavor)

Toast the waffle. Spread with cream cheese and then the fruit spread. Cut into 3 to 4 "sticks" to eat.

Tuna Salad Snack

1 small tomato
2 ounces chunk light tuna in water, drained
1 tablespoon light ranch dressing

Cut out tomato stem, then cut tomato into four wedges, leaving them connected at the bottom of the tomato. Place tuna in a small bowl. Add dressing and mix to combine. Spoon tuna on top of tomato wedges.

Chocolate Yogurt Sundae

½ of a 6-ounce container Chobani Greek nonfat vanilla yogurt
¼ cup Chocolate Cheerios cereal

Place yogurt in a small bowl. Top with cereal.

Berry Bagel

½ cup ripe sliced strawberries
1 teaspoon sugar
½ Thomas' 100% Whole Wheat Bagel Thins bagel

Place strawberries and sugar in a small bowl. Use the back of a fork to lightly mash strawberries. Be careful not to mash so much that they become liquid. You want them to be like a spreadable jam. Toast bagel. Spread strawberry mixture on top.

Tomato-Basil Melt

½ of a Thomas' Light Multi-Grain English muffin
1 small Roma tomato (Italian plum tomato), sliced
2-3 fresh basil leaves
2 tablespoons shredded mozzarella cheese

Preheat oven to 400°F. Toast English muffin half. Top with tomato, basil, and mozzarella cheese. Bake for 4 to 5 minutes, or until cheese is melted.

Health Tip: Two compounds in basil—*orientin* and *vicenin*—are potent inhibitors of free radicals, the cell-hurting molecules that are a main cause of aging and chronic disease.

Cinnamon Bagel with Orange Spread

½ Thomas' Cinnamon Raisin Bagel Thins bagel
1 tablespoon reduced-fat cream cheese
2 teaspoons orange juice
¼–½ teaspoon grated orange peel

Toast bagel. Place cream cheese in a small bowl. Add orange juice and orange peel. Mix well, then spread on toasted bagel half.

Health Tip: Studies in *Nutrition Research*[20] and the *American Journal of Clinical Nutrition*[21] show orange juice can lower LDL cholesterol and raise good (HDL) cholesterol.

Open-Faced Cucumber Sandwich

½ Arnold Sandwich Thin
¼ cup low-fat cottage cheese
¼ cucumber, peeled and cut into thin slices
Dash lemon-pepper seasoning or salt

Toast sandwich thin. Top with cottage cheese and cucumber slices. Sprinkle with lemon-pepper seasoning or salt.

Health Tip: Studies link regular intake of cottage cheese and other calcium-rich dairy products with balanced blood sugar, lower blood pressure, less weight gain, and a smaller waistline.

Strawberries and Cream Toast

½ Arnold Sandwich Thins Roll
1 wedge Laughing Cow Smooth Sensations Cream Cheese
    Spread (⅓ Less Fat), Strawberries & Cream flavor
1 strawberry, sliced

Toast the sandwich thin. Spread cream cheese on top, then top with strawberry slices.

Almond-Cherry Smoothie

1 cup Blue Diamond Almond Breeze unsweetened chocolate almond milk

½ cup frozen dark sweet cherries

1 cup ice

Place almond milk, cherries, and ice in a blender. Blend until combined.

Health Tip: Health is a bowl of cherries. Studies at Boston University School of Medicine show that cherries can help prevent gout (an increasingly common health problem) or prevent gout attacks if you already have the disease.[22] Other research shows cherries lower triglycerides and C-reactive protein, two risk factors for heart disease.[23] Cherries before bedtime can also improve sleep![24]

Ham and Cheese Spirals

½ teaspoon mustard

1 (1-ounce) slice lean deli ham

1 leaf butterhead (Bibb) lettuce

1 (1-ounce) mozzarella cheese stick

Spread mustard on ham. Place lettuce on top. Put cheese stick in the center of the lettuce. Roll up from one side to the other. Cut the roll-up into 2 to 3 pieces to serve.

Health Tip: A little mustard goes a long way toward better health. The mustard plant is in the cancer-fighting crucifer family, which includes broccoli, Brussels sprouts, kale, and cabbage. And the mustard seed contains concentrated amounts of the same anticancer compounds found in those greens.

Cinnamon Tortilla Strips

1 small (fajita-size) Mission Carb Balance whole wheat tortilla

1 teaspoon cinnamon-sugar seasoning

Preheat oven to 350°F. Place tortilla on a cutting board. Spray one side with nonstick cooking spray. Sprinkle cinnamon sugar evenly over tortilla. Cut into 4 to 5 strips. Transfer strips to baking sheet. Bake for 6 to 9 minutes, or until strips are crisp and lightly browned.

Preparation Tip: If you don't have cinnamon-sugar seasoning, combine 1 teaspoon sugar with 1/8 teaspoon cinnamon.

Taco Dip with Peppers

1/4 cup reduced-fat sour cream
1/2 teaspoon taco seasoning
1 tablespoon jarred salsa
1 green sweet pepper, seeded and cut into thin strips

Place sour cream, taco seasoning, and salsa in a small bowl. Mix to combine. Serve with green pepper strips.

Crackers with Vegetable Spread

1 tablespoon Kraft Philadelphia Garden Vegetable 1/3 Less Fat cream cheese
2 Wasa Light Rye crispbreads
1 tablespoon shredded carrot

Spread 1/2 tablespoon cream cheese on each crispbread. Top each with 1/2 tablespoon shredded carrot.

Health Tip: Finnish scientists call it the "Rye Factor"—the fact that blood sugar levels stay uniquely balanced after a meal that includes rye bread.[25]

Bananas with Crunchy Berry Topping

1/2 banana
1 tablespoon Chobani Greek nonfat vanilla yogurt
1/4 cup Kellogg's Special K Red Berries cereal

Cut the banana in half lengthwise and place on a plate, cut side up. Spread ½ tablespoon yogurt on the cut surface of each banana. Top each with 2 tablespoons of the cereal.

Berries with Fruit Dip

3 tablespoons plain nonfat Greek yogurt
2 teaspoons Polaner All Fruit spread (any flavor)
6 medium strawberries, hulled

Place yogurt and fruit spread in small bowl. Mix to combine, then use as a dip for the strawberries.

Health Tip: Adding strawberries to your diet for eight weeks decreases total and LDL cholesterol, report scientists from Oklahoma State University in *Nutrition Research*.[26]

Turkey-Lettuce Rolls

3 (1-ounce) slices deli turkey breast
3 dill pickle spears
3 small leaves of lettuce

Wrap each slice of turkey around a pickle spear; then wrap lettuce around the turkey.

Sweet-and-Salty Snack Mix

1 cup Skinny Pop popcorn
11 Pepperidge Farm Original Goldfish crackers
⅓ cup Berry Berry Kix Cereal

Place popcorn, crackers, and cereal in a medium bowl. Toss to combine.

Health Tip: As a snack, popcorn satisfies hunger and decreases appetite far better than potato chips, according to a study in *Nutrition Journal*.[27]

CHAPTER 5

Every-Other-Day Dieting, Without Lifting a Finger

Make your life super-simple: Heat up a frozen meal on Diet Day

When you think "frozen foods," do you still picture a TV dinner and its rubbery meat, mushy potatoes, and pebblelike peas? Well, if you haven't looked lately at what's behind the glass doors of your supermarket's frozen food section, you're in for a pleasant surprise.

Today's frozen entrées are twenty-first-century wonders of culinary ingenuity, designed for maximum flavor and nutrition. In fact, some of them were designed by famous chefs. Two examples: Bertolli frozen foods, created by Chef Rocco DiSpirito, author of the *New York Times* #1 bestseller *Now Eat*

This!; and Barefoot Contessa Sauté Dinners for Two, created by Ina Garten, star of the *Barefoot Contessa* program on the Food Network.

You can choose from ethnic cuisines, like Italian, Mexican, and Chinese. You can dine on casual fare like pizza or buffalo wings or on classic American favorites like meat loaf or macaroni and cheese. If you're vegetarian, you can enjoy tasty meat substitutes. You can even eat organic foods.

And here's the really good news for Every-Other-Day dieters: you can find *hundreds* of frozen food entrées of 400 calories or less, well within the limits of the 500 calories of Diet Day. (The entrées we have chosen are typically 400 calories or less, because it's good to leave room for a 100-calorie snack; that allows you to eat twice during Diet Day.)

Bottom line: Eating a 400-calorie (or less) frozen entrée for lunch or dinner is probably the easiest and surest way to handle Diet Day in the Every-Other-Day Diet and to lose all the weight you want to lose, as quickly as possible.

- *Easiest*, because all you have to do is stick the entrée in the microwave. In the case of frozen "skillet meals," you'll spend 10 minutes or so at the stove.
- *Surest*, because you'll know without a doubt that the meal you're eating is within the calorie limits of Diet Day.

In many of my studies we provided participants with frozen entrées, and we found they *really* enjoyed using frozen meals as a simple and convenient way to control their calories on Diet Day. In fact, once the study was over, they often went to the supermarket looking for exactly the same entrées and discovered, to their delight, that there was an entire world of choices available.

In this chapter you will find a range of tasty selections, which we put together with help from our recipe developer, Stephanie Karpinske, MS, RD, a registered dietitian, nutritionist, and cookbook author.

We've organized the frozen foods into four categories:

- Classic American cuisine
- Low calorie, high flavor
- Organic, natural, and vegetarian
- Ethnic cuisine

Within each of these categories, we describe the top brands and then offer several Diet Day Delights from that brand, entrées we think you'll really like. We used several criteria to choose those brands and the entrées within them, including the following:

- *A range of calories* under the Diet Day limit of 500. You'll find entrées from 100 to 490 calories. If your entrée is low enough, have another!
- *Variety*, so you don't become bored by Diet Day.
- *Flavor*, for mealtime enjoyment.
- *Hearty and light meals.* We wanted you to have a choice of heartier, heavier dishes for the cold months of winter, like meat loaf and mashed potatoes, and lighter dishes for spring and summer, like pasta.

We've also included a Two-Month Diet Day Meal Plan, which provides a selection of 30 frozen entrées for 30 Diet Days. If you want to diet longer than two months, just repeat the plan after you reach Day 60. If you decide to manage Diet Day using frozen foods, following the Meal Plan in this chapter isn't a must. The choices of entrées are just suggestions. If you like, choose your own entrées, as long as they're 500 calories or less.

Since the entrées are less than 500 calories, every Diet Day can include one or more snacks. To make your snack choices super-simple, we've included an extensive list of snacks from 50 to 160 calories, organized by calorie level (50 calories, 90 to 100 calories, 100 calories, etc.). Just match the snack to the entrée. For example, if the entrée is 400 calories, choose a 100-calorie snack. Or if the entrée is 350 calories, choose a 150-calorie snack.

With this chapter you never need to rigorously count calories, because they're counted for you. Follow the Two-Month Diet Day Meal Plan, and you'll never exceed 500 calories on Diet Day. *And* you never need to figure out what to eat, because we've made a tasty choice for your entrée and provided a big list of snacks that match. All you have to do is lose weight, and with the Two-Month Diet Day Meal Plan, weight loss is virtually automatic.

MAXIMIZE YOUR MICROWAVE

When you follow the Two-Month Diet Day Meal Plan, you're going to be using the microwave oven a lot. Maybe you'll even use that old microwave oven at the office when you cook lunch. Although cooking in a microwave is pretty simple, there are a few key tips for making sure your food is cooked evenly and safely.

Don't just heat—cook. Frozen foods should be *cooked*, not just heated. That's because an undercooked beef tip or chicken breast can harbor salmonella, the bacteria that cause food poisoning. Your best bet: buy a meat thermometer and check meat to make sure it's truly done. Chicken should be at least 170°F and beef from 145°F (medium) to 170°F (well done).

Pay attention to wattage. The power output of microwave ovens typically ranges from 600 to 1,200 watts; a higher wattage cooks more quickly and evenly. But wattage decreases as ovens age. So the entrée's package may say to microwave the entrée for 3 minutes, but if you're using a 10- or 20-year-old microwave, you may need to microwave the entrée for 5 minutes for it to cook thoroughly. Again, use your food thermometer to make sure meat is *cooked*.

The microwave's wattage is on the front of the unit or inside the door. Can't find the wattage of your microwave? Boil a cup of water, timing the boiling point. A 700-watt microwave boils water in 2 minutes and 30 seconds; a 1,000-watt oven boils water in 1 minute and 45 seconds; a 600-watt oven, in 2 minutes and 55 seconds. (For a chart that matches boiling points and wattages, ranging from 300 to 1,625 watts, see the web page www.microwavecookingforone.com/Charts/Wattage.html, at the site of Marie T. Smith, author of *Microwave Cooking for One*.)

(continued)

Don't use the preset button. Your microwave may have a suggested preprogrammed setting, such as "Frozen Meal." Don't use it. Follow the directions on the package, cooking your meal for the designated time.

Check all the directions and follow them. If the directions on the packaging say to turn the food halfway through the cooking time, or lift the cover, or not to uncover the food, follow those directions. Your meal is more likely to taste as it was intended to taste: good, not undercooked or overcooked.

Don't cook two meals at once. Unless the packaging says it's okay to do so, don't put two microwave meals in the oven at the same time—they use more energy and won't cook as evenly.

Cook in the packaging supplied by the manufacturer. Don't transfer the food to another dish or container for cooking. You're likely to find the food doesn't cook as well; for example, a crispy crust might end up soggy.

Stand back a foot or two. The waves in microwaves are a form of electromagnetic radiation, similar to the radiation emitted by your television set, computer monitor, hair dryer, air conditioner, and vacuum cleaner. Are those waves dangerous? Many environmental experts say no. Other experts, such as David Carpenter, MD, director of the Institute for Health and the Environment at the University at Albany, New York, say it's better to be cautious—that even the low levels of electromagnetic radiation emitted by appliances might damage cells.

Dr. Carpenter's advice: Stand a few feet away from the front of the microwave while your food is cooking. Standing just 1 foot away reduces the radiation from 200 to 40 milligauss (mG); standing four feet away reduces it to 2 mG.

DIET DAY FROZEN MEALS

Classic American Cuisine

Banquet

Since 1953, Banquet has been helping people make quick and easy meals with the company's line of frozen pot pies and classic TV dinners. Today, their lineup still includes a wide variety of treasured favorites, like fried chicken. Many of the dinners come with a side dish and small dessert, making them a complete and satisfying meal.

Diet Day Delights:
- Swedish Meatballs (440 calories)
- Original Fried Chicken Meal (440 calories)
- Homestyle Charbroiled Patty Meal with Noodles (310 calories)

Birds Eye

You know them best for their wide assortment of frozen vegetables, but Birds Eye also makes Voila!, a line of skillet meals that are ready in 10 to 15 minutes. These bagged meals come in two sizes: regular and family. The regular size makes three 1⅔-cup servings; the family size makes six 1½-cup servings. The calories in these meals are very low: you can increase the serving size and still be within your limit for Diet Day.

Diet Day Delights:

- Voila! Garlic Shrimp (230 calories)
- Voila! Beef & Broccoli Stir Fry (210 calories)
- Voila! Three Cheese Chicken (210 calories)

Boston Market

Craving comfort food? Make a reservation at the Boston Market. You can re-create this restaurant's home-style meals in your own kitchen with one of their many frozen entrées. Just be sure to check the Nutrition Facts panel, because some entrées exceed 500 calories.

Diet Day Delights:

- Beef Steak and Noodles (460 calories)
- Country Fried Chicken (450 calories)
- Beef Pot Roast (390 calories)
- Turkey Breast Medallions with Stuffing (380 calories)

California Pizza Kitchen

If you love this chain's pizza, make it at home with one of their many frozen options. To make sure the calories work for Diet Day, check the label and eat the right portion size.

For example, one-third of the Signature Pepperoni pizza is 380 calories. Or choose one of the small, individual-sized pizzas. *Tip:* Look for the thin-crust variety—you'll get more pizza for your calories!

Diet Day Delights:

- Small Crispy Thin Crust Margherita (430 calories)
- Small Crispy Thin Crust Pizza Hawaiian Recipe (380 calories)
- Signature Pepperoni (340 calories for ⅓ of the pizza)
- Crispy Thin Crust BBQ Recipe Chicken (310 calories for ⅓ of the pizza)
- Crispy Thin Crust Garlic Chicken (280 calories for ⅓ of the pizza)

Gorton's

This brand is known for their fish sticks but offers much more. Choose from a range of fish and seafood entrées, including beer-battered shrimp, seasoned fish fillets, and shrimp scampi. Serve with a frozen vegetable and you'll have a complete meal.

Diet Day Delights:

- Premium Haddock Fish Sticks (250 calories for 4 fish sticks)
- Crispy HomeStyle Shrimp (240 calories for 5 shrimp)
- Crispy Beer Batter Shrimp (240 calories for 5 shrimp)
- Lemon Butter Shrimp Scampi (240 calories for 12 shrimp)

Jimmy Dean

For scientific consistency, my studies on EOD dieting always use lunch as the sole meal on Diet Day; I think that's the ideal approach for EOD dieters, since it's the approach that has been proven to work. In this book, however, I'm including dinner as an option, because you might want to eat with your spouse or family.

But what if you're a person who loves eating *breakfast*, and forgoing breakfast every Diet Day feels like too much of a sacrifice? Well, have breakfast for lunch or dinner with frozen entrées from Jimmy Dean.

For a super-fast meal, try one of the heat-and-eat bowls or a take-and-go sandwich or quesadilla. Other options include omelets, pancakes, and skillet meals. Calories vary, so check the package for calories per serving before buying. *Tip:* The Jimmy Dean Delights line is lower in calories than their traditional products.

Diet Day Delights:
- Bacon Breakfast Bowl (430 calories)
- Delights Turkey Sausage Quesadilla (250 calories per serving; box contains 2 servings)
- Delights Honey Wheat Flatbread: Turkey, Egg & Cheese (250 calories)
- Delights Turkey Sausage Breakfast Bowl (240 calories)

Marie Callender's

These restaurant-inspired meals are lightened-up versions of favorite comfort foods, such as chicken pot pie, roast beef with mashed potatoes, and meat loaf and gravy. They're so good you may think you're cheating on the Every-Other-Day Diet—but you're not! All the meals from this brand are under 500 calories.

Diet Day Delights:

- Country Fried Pork Chop and Gravy (460 calories)
- Chunky Chicken & Noodles (440 calories)
- Creamy Parmesan Chicken Pot Pie (420 calories)
- Comfort Bakes: Cheddar & Bacon Potato Bake (400 calories)
- Steak & Roasted Potatoes (350 calories)
- Honey Roasted Turkey Breast (350 calories)

Stouffer's

You're sure to find something you like with the many offerings from Stouffer's. Choose from old-fashioned entrées like Chicken a la King to modern favorites like flatbread sandwiches. You can buy meals that make one or two servings or enough for the entire family.

Diet Day Delights:

- Satisfying Servings Bourbon Steak Tips (490 calories)
- Steak Cheddar Mushroom Flatbread Melt (390 calories)
- Signature Classics Smoked Turkey Club Panini (380 calories)
- French Bread Pizza Grilled Vegetables Pizza (340 calories for ½ of the package)
- Satisfying Servings Stuffed Green Peppers (300 calories for 2 peppers)

Trader Joe's

When my kitchen was being remodeled and I had no working refrigerator or freezer, I began buying two frozen food entrées on the way home from work and heating them in the microwave (the one kitchen appliance that was still working) for myself and my husband. (This was several years before my son was born.) We tried many different brands, and I have to say that my favorite was Trader Joe's. They were inexpensive, didn't overdo it on the calories, and were tasty, with a minimum amount of artificial ingredients.

If you decide to shop at this specialty grocer, you'll find a wide range of choices in the frozen food aisle, including comfort foods, ethnic entrées, and vegetarian meals. And the frozen entrées aren't frozen in time: Trader Joe's adds new or seasonal products throughout the year, so check their in-store flyer to see what's available.

Diet Day Delights:
- Shepherd's Pie with Meat (380 calories for 2 cups)
- Chicken Lasagna (330 calories/serving)
- Chicken Tikka Masala (300 calories). This is my personal favorite, and also the favorite of the blog *What's Good at Trader Joe's*, which enthuses, "It tastes just as authentic as the food from the best Indian restaurants I've been to."
- Reduced Guilt Roasted Vegetable Pizza (250 calories)

Tyson Foods

Tyson offers lots of options for chicken lovers, including breaded products and preseasoned boneless, skinless chicken breasts. Their products are typically sold in large bags, so if you're preparing food for you and your family, you can make as many pieces as you need. For an easy dinner, bake some chicken in the oven, then microwave a frozen vegetable for a side.

Diet Day Delights:
- Chicken Nuggets (430 calories for 8 nuggets)
- Spicy Chicken Breast Patties (400 calories for 2 patties)
- Fully Cooked Mesquite Chicken Breast (400 calories for 2 chicken breasts)
- Chicken Breast Tenders (384 calories for 8 tenders)

Low Calorie, High Flavor

Healthy Choice

This brand is a standout when it comes to variety, offering everything from traditional classics to ethnic foods. Every item in their Complete Meals line includes an entrée, side dish, and dessert. They also have one-dish meals under their Café Steamers and Baked Entrée lines. And their 100% Natural line offers steamed meals that contain no preservatives.

Diet Day Delights:
- Complete Meals: Chicken Parmigiana (340 calories)
- Café Steamers: Barbecue Seasoned Steak with Red Potatoes (320 calories)
- Pumpkin Squash Ravioli (310 calories)

Lean Cuisine

While we were researching and writing this chapter, my coauthor Bill was exploring the frozen foods section of a local supermarket and saw a middle-aged man (without much extra fat around his middle) loading his shopping cart with Lean Cuisine entrées; he decided to conduct a "man in the aisle" interview, asking him why he favored Lean Cuisine.

His response? "It has the most variety, tastes the best, and it helped me lose weight and keep it off."

I'm not surprised by what this shopper had to say. Lean Cuisine is one the favorite frozen food brands of the participants in my studies. And "variety" is an understatement. With nearly 100 entrées, the brand is divided into four recipe collections: Culinary, Spa, Market, and Simple Favorites. And for salad lovers, Lean Cuisine recently introduced Salad Additions—just add fresh greens for a complete, hearty salad meal. Because it's a favorite of those on the EOD Diet, I've included a bigger list of top choices.

Diet Day Delights:
- Jumbo Rigatoni with Meatballs (420 calories)
- Roasted Honey Chicken (320 calories)
- Tuscan-Style Vegetable Lasagna (320 calories)
- French Bread Pepperoni Pizza (310 calories)
- Tortilla Crusted Fish with Rice, Poblano Peppers, and Corn (300 calories)
- Cranberry & Chicken Salad (from Salad Additions

collection; 280 calories plus the calories in the salad greens at about 10 calories/cup)
- Salmon with Basil (250 calories)

Lean Pockets

These low-calorie cousins of the Hot Pockets brand are great for a portable heat-and-eat meal. And although you can eat them with a fork, they're just as easily eaten like a sandwich. Plus, there's plenty of choices, including pockets made with pretzel bread or whole grains. There's even a line of breakfast entrées.

Diet Day Delights:
- Lean Pockets Pretzel Bread Sandwiches: Grilled Chicken Jalapeño Cheddar (280 calories)
- Lean Pockets Culinary Creations (made with whole-grain flour): Spinach Artichoke Chicken (250 calories)
- Lean Pockets Culinary Creations: Grilled Chicken, Mushroom & Wild Rice (250 calories)

Note: Calories are per Lean Pocket, and each package contains 2 pockets.

Michelina's Lean Gourmet

This popular brand of frozen dinners also offers low-calorie options in its Lean Gourmet line. You'll find entrées for breakfast, lunch, and dinner, as well as a few snack options, some of which are hearty enough for a meal.

Diet Day Delights:

- Shrimp Scampi (290 calories)
- Beef Supreme (290 calories)
- Macaroni and Cheese with Jalapeño Peppers (270 calories)
- Creamy Rigatoni with Broccoli and Chicken (270 calories)
- Shrimp with Pasta and Vegetables (260 calories)

Smart Ones

This Weight Watchers' brand of frozen food entrées includes something for everyone. You'll find comfort foods, handheld meals, and nutrient-packed entrées, as well as large-portion dinners that have more protein and whole grains to keep you feeling full. Smart Ones also has a line of breakfast entrées and desserts.

Diet Day Delights:

- Smart Anytime: Savory Steak & Ranch Grilled Flat-bread (330 calories)
- Smart Anytime: Pepperoni Pizza Minis (280 calories)
- Smart Beginnings: French Toast with Turkey Sausage (280 calories)
- Smart Creations: Chicken Mesquite (250 calories)
- Classic Favorites: Broccoli & Cheddar Roasted Potatoes (240 calories)

Organic, Natural, and Vegetarian

Amy's

All of Amy's frozen entrées are organic, vegetarian, and free of additives and preservatives. They're also boredom-free: Amy's wide variety includes Mexican, Chinese, and Indian fare, as well as American classics like pot pies and single-serve pizzas. My personal favorite is Macaroni & Cheese. Most of the entrées are already low in calories, but Amy's also offers a Light and Lean line that has even fewer calories.

Diet Day Delights:
- Broccoli Pot Pie (460 calories)
- Indian Mattar Paneer (370 calories)
- Teriyaki Wrap (310 calories)
- Brown Rice, Black-Eyed Peas & Veggies Bowl (290 calories)
- Light & Lean Italian Vegetable Pizza (280 calories)
- Spinach Feta in a Pocket Wrap (260 calories)

Boca Foods

When you crave a burger but don't want all the calories, check out the many meatless options from Boca. You can't go wrong with their basic hamburger or cheeseburger, but Boca also makes vegetable patties and meatless chicken (chik'n) patties. All of the burgers and patties are so low in calories that you'll have plenty of room to add a bun, some tasty toppers, and a side dish—maybe even dessert!

Diet Day Delights:

- Spicy Chik'n Patty (160 calories)
- All American Flame Grilled Burger (120 calories)
- Savory Mushroom Mozzarella Veggie Patty (110 calories)
- Cheeseburger (100 calories)

Gardein

The goal of this brand is to deliver meatless products that taste just like meat—and they've succeeded. From texture to flavor, these entrées—riblets, sliders, cutlets, and the like—might even trick a Texan. Heat up some frozen vegetables or toss together a salad to make a complete meal.

Diet Day Delights:

- Southern BBQ Riblets (300 calories for 2 riblets with sauce)
- The Ultimate Beefless Sliders (300 calories for 2 sliders)
- Lightly Breaded Turk'y Cutlet (250 calories for 2 cutlets)
- Classic Style Buffalo Wings (180 calories for 8 wings)

Kashi

If you prefer brown rice to white rice and whole wheat to white flour, try this brand, which offers foods containing Kashi's special blend of seven whole grains. Kashi includes a line of tasty, one-serving pizzas (with whole-grain crust, of course). And they recently came out with 2-serving Steam Meals, a line of frozen meals in a bag that cook in minutes in the microwave. (The steam keeps the veggies crisp and keeps the whole-grain pasta from being overcooked.)

Diet Day Delights:

- Mayan Harvest Bake (340 calories)
- Black Bean Mango (340 calories)
- Steam Meals Chicken and Chipotle Barbecue (310 calories for half of the bag)
- Lemongrass Coconut Chicken (300 calories)
- Thin-Crust Pizza Mushroom Trio & Spinach (250 calories for ⅓ of the pizza)

MorningStar Farms

You might not realize you're eating vegetarian when you dine on the meatless options from MorningStar Farms. They make an assortment of meatless burgers, vegetarian "chik'n" patties and nuggets, veggie hot dogs—even veggie corn dogs.

Diet Day Delights:

- Chik'n Nuggets (380 calories for 8 nuggets)
- Three Bean Chili with Grillers Crumbles (340 calories for 2 cups)
- Veggie Corn Dogs (300 calories for 2 corn dogs)
- Grillers ¼ Pounder (250 calories; add a small bun for an additional 110 to 120 calories)

Newman's Own Skillet Meals for 2

If microwaved food isn't your thing, try one of these super-easy skillet meals, ready in just 10 minutes—just put it in the skillet, gently stir while cooking, and serve. Featuring all-natural ingredients, each bag serves 2, so you can share the other half or save it for another meal. An added bonus: the company donates its profits to charity.

Diet Day Delights:

- Beef Bolognese (390 calories for ½ of the package)
- Chicken Florentine and Farfalle (370 calories for ½ of the package)
- Garlic Chicken, Vegetables and Farfalle (300 calories for ½ of the package)

Ethnic Cuisine

Bertolli (Italian)

You might think of olive oil or pasta sauce when you think of Bertolli, but you can also find this brand in the freezer aisle. They make a line of hearty frozen soups (Meal Soups), Italian entrées (Classic Meals), and meals based on the heart-healthy Mediterranean Diet (Mediterranean Style Meals). Keep in mind that these frozen meals make 2 servings, not 1. Also note that not all their meals are low-calorie, so check the label to make sure you're within your Diet Day quota of calories.

Diet Day Delights:

- Classic Meals for Two: Roasted Chicken & Linguine (410 calories for ½ of the package)
- Mediterranean Style Meals, for Two: Steak, Rigatoni & Portobello Mushrooms (390 calories for ½ of the package)

- Meal Soups: Ricotta and Lobster Ravioli in a Seafood Bisque (380 calories for ½ of the package)
- Mediterranean Style Meals for Two: Garlic Shrimp, Penne & Cherry Tomatoes (340 calories for ½ of the package)

El Monterey (Mexican)

This brand offers frozen burritos and chimichangas, many of which are low enough in calories to eat as a snack on Diet Day. Their tamales are also a good low-calorie option. Most El Monterey burritos and chimichangas are available in single portions, a plus if you like variety.

Diet Day Delights:
- Butcher Wrapped Shredded Beef Steak & Cheese Burrito (450 calories)
- Beef & Bean Burrito (370 calories)
- All Natural Chicken & Monterey Jack Cheese Chimichanga (280 calories)
- Bean & Cheese Burrito (190 calories)

InnovAsian Cuisine (Chinese)

Skip the Chinese takeout and try an entrée from InnovAsian Cuisine: pop it in the microwave and your meal will be ready in 5 minutes. These dinners have far fewer calories than the same dish in a Chinese restaurant, leaving you plenty of room for a snack. Servings per package vary on these meals, so measure out your portions. The nutrition info on the label is based on a 1-cup serving.

Diet Day Delights:

- Sweet & Sour Chicken (430 calories for 1 cup)
- Caramelized Ginger Pork (270 calories for 1 cup)
- Spicy Beef & Broccoli (160 calories for 1 cup)

Mrs. T's (Polish)

Attention, carb lovers: you're going to adore Mrs. T's Pierogies, a tasty combo of pasta and potatoes. There are several varieties to choose from, including a sweet potato pierogi made with whole grains. Each box contains several pierogies, so share a few with your family or save the extras for another Diet Day.

Diet Day Delights:

- Sweet Potato Pierogies (380 calories for 6 pierogies)
- Potato, Broccoli & Cheddar Pierogies (380 for 6 pierogies)
- Potato Spinach & Feta Pierogies (360 calories for 8 pierogies)

P.F. Chang's Home Menu (Chinese)

Now you can serve some of the rice and noodle dishes from this popular restaurant at home. The meals serve 2 and are ready in 13 minutes or less. But check the calories before buying—some meals push you past your limit for Diet Day.

Diet Day Delights:

- General Chang's Chicken (400 calories for ½ of the package)
- Shrimp Lo Mein (400 calories for ½ of the package)
- Ginger Chicken and Broccoli (320 calories for ½ of the package)

Pagoda Express (Chinese)

This brand's lineup of frozen meals includes some traditional favorites, like Orange Chicken. Each meal makes 2 servings and cooks up in the microwave in minutes. For some lower calorie meals, such as Beef & Broccoli, you could eat 2 servings and still not exceed your Diet Day calories.

Diet Day Delights:
- Orange Chicken (270 calories for 1 cup)
- Beef & Broccoli (240 calories for 1 cup)
- Teriyaki Beef (220 calories for 1 cup)
- Spicy Garlic Chicken (210 calories for 1 cup)

YOUR TWO-MONTH (SUPER-CONVENIENT, SUPER-EASY) DIET DAY MEAL PLAN

Is there anything easier than microwaving a frozen entrée for your Diet Day meal? Yes! Choosing all the entrées recommended in our Two-Month Diet Day Meal Plan. By following the plan, you won't have to make *any* mealtime decisions on Diet Day. Just eat the meal suggested and then choose a snack from our Mix-and-Match Snack list at the end of the chapter, combining the entrée's calories with the snacks to match your daily calorie goal. *Example:* If the entrée has 380 calories, you'll select a snack of 120 calories for a total of 500 calories.

But don't worry too much if you exceed the 500 calories by 25 to 50 calories—for example, if you eat a 400-calorie entrée and choose a 120-calorie snack. What's important is that on most

Diet Days you are very near your 500-calorie goal, and you rarely exceed that amount by more than 50 calories. Ready to start the Every-Other-Day Diet today?

Diet Day 1

Entrée: Lean Cuisine Pepperoni Pizza (380 calories)
Snack: 120-calorie snack

Diet Day 3

Entrée: InnovAsian Caramelized Ginger Pork (270 calories for 1 cup)
Snack: A 230-calorie entrée; or 230 calories of snacks

Diet Day 5

Entrée: Marie Callender's Comfort Bakes: Cheddar and Bacon Potato Bake (400 calories)
Snack: 100-calorie snack

Diet Day 7

Entrée: Lean Cuisine Chicken Club Panini (360 calories)
Snack: 140-calorie snack

Diet Day 9

Entrée: Birds Eye Voila! Garlic Shrimp (230 calories)
Snack: A 270-calorie entrée; or 270 calories of snacks

Diet Day 11

Entrée: Newman's Own Beef Bolognese (390 calories for
½ of the package)
Snack: 110-calorie snack

Diet Day 13

Entrée: Boston Market Country Fried Chicken
(450 calories)
Snack: 50-calorie snack

Diet Day 15

Entrée: Jimmy Dean Bacon Breakfast Bowl: Bacon, Eggs,
Potatoes and Cheddar Cheese (410 calories)
Snack: 90-calorie snack

Diet Day 17

Entrée: Healthy Choice Chicken Parmigiana
(340 calories)
Snack: 160 calories of snacks

Diet Day 19

Entrée: Amy's Broccoli Pot Pie (460 calories)
Snack: 50-calorie snack

Diet Day 21

Entrée: Gorton's Premium Haddock Fish Sticks
(250 calories for 4 fish sticks)
Snack: Another 250-calorie entrée; or 250 calories of
snacks

Diet Day 23

Entrée: El Monterey Butcher Wrapped Shredded Beef
Steak & Cheese Burrito (450 calories)
Snack: 50-calorie snack

Diet Day 25

Entrée: California Pizza Kitchen Small Crispy Thin Crust
Pizza Hawaiian Recipe (380 calories)
Snack: 120-calorie snack

Diet Day 27

Entrée: Pagoda Express Orange Chicken (270 calories for
1 cup)
Snack: 130-calorie snack

Diet Day 29

Entrée: Stouffer's Steak Cheddar Mushroom Flatbread Melt
(390 calories)
Snack: 110-calorie snack

Diet Day 31

Entrée: Tyson Chicken Breast Tenders (384 calories for
8 tenders)
Snack: 110-calorie snack

Diet Day 33

Entrée: Boca All American Flame Grilled Burger (120
calories plus 110-calorie hamburger bun = 230 calories)
Snack: A 270-calorie entrée; or 270 calories of snacks

Diet Day 35

Entrée: P.F. Chang's Shrimp Lo Mein (400 calories for ½ of
the package)
Snack: 100-calorie snack

Diet Day 37

Entrée: Mrs. T's Potato, Broccoli & Cheddar Pierogies
(380 calories for 6 pierogies)
Snack: 120-calorie snack

Diet Day 39

Entrée: Lean Pockets Pretzel Bread Sandwiches:
Roasted Turkey with Bacon and Reduced-Fat Cheese
(280 calories)
Snack: A 220-calorie entrée; or 220 calories of snacks

Diet Day 41

Entrée: Trader Joe's Chicken Lasagna (330 calories per serving)

Snack: 170 calories of snacks

Diet Day 43

Entrée: Smart Ones Smart Beginnings French Toast with Turkey Sausage (280 calories)

Snack: A 220-calorie entrée; or 220 calories of snacks

Diet Day 45

Entrée: Gardein Southern BBQ Riblets (300 calories for 2 riblets with sauce)

Snack: A 200-calorie entrée; or 200 calories of snacks

Diet Day 47

Entrée: Banquet Homestyle Charbroiled Patty Meal with Noodles (310 calories)

Snack: 190 calories of snacks

Diet Day 49

Entrée: Lean Cuisine Roasted Honey Chicken (320 calories)

Snack: 180 calories of snacks

Diet Day 51

Entrée: Michelina's Lean Gourmet Macaroni and Cheese
with Jalapeño Peppers (270 calories)
Snack: A 230-calorie entrée; or 230 calories of snacks

Diet Day 53

Entrée: Marie Callender's Country Fried Pork Chop and
Gravy (460 calories)
Snack: 50-calorie snack

Diet Day 55

Entrée: MorningStar Farms Veggie Corn Dogs
(300 calories for 2 corn dogs)
Snack: 200 calories of snacks

Diet Day 57

Entrée: Bertolli Classic Meals for Two: Tuscan Style
Braised Beef with Gold Potatoes (310 calories for ½ of
the package)
Snack: 190 calories of snacks

Diet Day 59

Entrée: Kashi Steam Meals Chicken and Chipotle
Barbecue (310 calories for ½ of the bag)
Snack: 190 calories of snacks

MIX-AND-MATCH SNACKS

Diet Day consists of a main meal—either lunch or dinner—and one or more snacks. Remember: you can eat *anything* you want, low-fat or high-fat, as long as you don't exceed your daily total of 500 calories. The snacks below are organized by calories; simply find a snack you like that matches the amount of calories in your Diet Day entrée so the total is 500.

And remember, too, these are just examples, for your convenience. Feel free to eat any other snack that doesn't take you over your Diet Day calories. That includes the delicious, 100-calorie snacks you'll find in chapter 4, "Diet Day Recipes—Quick, Easy, and Delicious," which offers 28 recipes for 100-calorie snacks.

50-calorie snacks (for 450-calorie entrées)

- 1 cup diced watermelon
- 2 small plums
- 1 small peach
- 1 medium kiwi fruit
- ¾ cup whole grapes
- 7 dry-roasted almonds

90- to 100-calorie snacks (for 400- to 410-calorie entrées)

- 1 medium apple
- 1 large orange

- 2 cups diced watermelon (1 cup diced watermelon is 50 calories)
- Yoplait Light yogurt, 1 container, Banana Cream Pie and other flavors
- Kellogg's Special K Cereal Bars, Blueberry flavor
- 1 Quaker Chewy Granola Bar
- 3 small plums
- 2 small peaches
- 1 medium banana
- 2 medium kiwi fruit
- 1½ cups whole grapes (¾ cup whole grapes is 50 calories)
- 15 dry-roasted almonds (7 dry-roasted almonds is 50 calories)
- Yoplait Greek 100, 1 container, Black Cherry and other flavors
- Kellogg's Special K Pastry Crisps, Strawberry and other flavors (2 crisps)
- 1 Kudos Milk Chocolate Granola Bar with Snickers (1 bar)
- Skinny Cow Mini Fudge Bars (2 bars)
- SnackWell's Devil's Food Cookies (2 cookies)
- Mott's Original Cinnamon Applesauce (single-serve container)
- Hunt's Snack Pack Vanilla Pudding (single-serve cup)
- Clif Mini bars, Oatmeal Raisin Walnut or other flavors (1 bar)

100-calorie snack packs (for 400-calorie entrées)

The snacks in this section are available in single-serve, 100-calorie packs. This isn't a complete list. That would require *The Every-Other-Day Diet*, volume 2. It's just meant to give you an idea of the range of 100-calorie snack packs on the shelves.

- Keebler Fudge Shoppe Mini Fudge Stripe Cookies
- Keebler Fudge Shoppe Fudge Grahams
- Sunshine Cheeze-It Baked Crackers
- Nabisco Chips Ahoy Cookies
- Nabisco Oreo Cookies
- Nabisco Lorna Doone Cookies
- Blue Diamond Almonds
- Baked Cheetos
- SmartFood Popcorn
- SunChips
- Ritz Snack Mix
- Snyder's of Hanover Mini Pretzels
- Lorna Doone Shortbread Cookie Crisps
- Chex Snack Mix (cheddar or chocolate caramel)
- Skinny Pop Popcorn
- Goldfish Crackers
- Jack Link's Beef Jerky
- Popchips
- Kellogg's Special K Fudge or Blondie Brownie Bites
- SnackWell's Popcorn
- SnackWell's Cookies
- Nabisco Cheese Nips Thin Crisps

110- to 120-calorie snacks (for 380- to 390-calorie entrées)

- Kellogg's Special K Protein Snack Bars, Dark Chocolate Granola (1 bar)
- Kellogg's Special K Cracker Chips, Sour Cream & Onion (27 chips)
- Newman's Own 94% Fat Free Microwave Popcorn (3½ cups popped)
- Orville Redenbacher's Smart Pop Butter Mini Bags microwave popcorn (per bag)
- Rold Gold Honey Wheat Braided Pretzel Twists (8 pretzels)
- Rold Gold Tiny Twists Pretzels (17 pretzels)
- Jell-O Butterscotch Pudding (single-serve cup)
- Luna Fiber bar, Chocolate Raspberry or Vanilla Blueberry flavors, 1 bar
- SnackWell's Creme Sandwich Cookies (2 cookies)
- 2 cups cubed cantaloupe or honeydew
- Kind Mini Bars, Cranberry Almond flavor
- Kind Vanilla Blueberry Clusters with Flax Seeds (⅓ cup)
- Baked Doritos Nacho Cheese Chips (15 chips)
- Baked Ruffles Cheddar & Sour Cream (1 ounce)
- Baked Lays Barbecue Potato Chips (1 ounce)
- Cracker Jack Original Caramel Coated Popcorn & Peanuts (½ cup)
- Snyder's of Hanover Pretzel Nibblers (16 nibblers)
- Kellogg's Special K Snack Crackers, Multigrain (24 crackers)

- Orville Redenbacher's Natural Simply Salted 50% Less Fat Microwave popcorn (5½ cups popped)

120- to 130-calorie snacks (for 370- to 380-calorie entrées)

- Fage Total 0% Yogurt, 1 single-serve container, Cherry Pomegranate and other flavors
- Dove Dark Chocolate Promises (3 pieces)
- Goldfish Pretzel crackers (43 pieces)
- Nabisco Wheat Thins Toasted Chips, Garden Valley Veggie (per serving)
- Nabisco Triscuit Thin Crisps, Four Cheese (per serving)
- Nabisco Reduced-Fat Cheese Nips, Cheddar (per serving)
- Jell-O Oreo Dirt Cup Pudding Mix-Ins (per single-serve container)
- Stacy's Toasted Garlic Bagel Chips (12 chips)
- Nabisco Teddy Graham's Chocolate Cookies (per serving, about 24 pieces)
- Nabisco Honey Graham Crackers (4 squares)

140- to 150-calorie snacks (for 355- to 360-calorie entrées)

- Quaker Popped Cheddar Cheese Snacks (per serving)
- Quaker Chewy Dipps Granola Bar (per bar)
- Quaker Soft-Baked bars (per bar)
- Smart Ones Chocolate Chip Cookie Dough Sundae
- Smart Ones Smart Delights Double Fudge Cake

- Chobani Greek Nonfat Yogurt, 6-ounce container, Blood Orange and other flavors
- Fage Total 1% Yogurt, 1 single-serve container, Blueberry and other flavors
- Goldfish Grahams, Vanilla Cupcake and Fudge Brownie flavors (35 pieces)
- Goldfish Crackers Pizza flavor (55 pieces)
- Goldfish Crackers Cheddar Made with Whole Grain (55 pieces)
- SunChips, Harvest Cheddar (1 ounce)
- Ruffles Reduced Fat Potato Chips (13 chips)
- Stacy's Cinnamon Sugar Pita Chips (7 chips)
- Orville Redenbacher's Smart Pop Kettle Corn microwave popcorn (7½ cups popped)
- Nabisco Wheat Thins, Original (per serving, approximately 16 pieces)
- Tostito's Bite-Size Tortilla Chips (24 chips)
- Doritos Taco Flavor Tortilla Chips (about 10 chips)
- Triscuit Baked Whole Grain Wheat Thin Crisps (for 16 crackers)

150- to 160-calorie snacks (for 340- to 350-calorie entrées)

- Smart Ones Smart Delights Key Lime Pie (1 dessert)
- Skinny Cow Low-Fat Ice Cream Cups, Chocolate Fudge Brownie and other flavors (1 cup)
- Skinny Cow Low-Fat Ice Cream Sandwich, Chocolate Peanut Butter and other flavors (1 sandwich)

- Skinny Cow Ice Cream Cone, Chocolate with Fudge and other flavors (1 cone)
- Dry-roasted peanuts (25 peanuts)
- Dry-roasted almonds (22 almonds)
- Cheetos Crunchy Cheese Flavored Snacks (21 pieces)
- Cheetos Puffs Simply Natural White Cheddar Cheese Flavored Snacks (32 pieces)
- Hershey's Special Dark Chocolate Nuggets with Almonds (3 pieces)
- Hershey's Simple Pleasures Dark Chocolate with Chocolate Crème (5 pieces)
- Jell-O German Chocolate Cake Pudding Mix-Ins (per single-serve cup)
- Quaker Instant Oatmeal flavored packet (1 single-serve packet)
- Lay's Original Potato Chips (15 chips)

CHAPTER 6

Every-Other-Day Dieting and Exercise

A powerful combo for faster weight loss, a leaner body, and a stronger heart

The Every-Other-Day Diet is strong medicine. It helps you shed pounds, a must for better health if you're overweight or obese. It can lower several risk factors for heart disease, including total and LDL cholesterol, triglycerides, and high blood pressure. It can balance blood sugar, helping prevent prediabetes and type 2 diabetes. And folks on the diet report a range of other health benefits, like more energy, clearer thinking, and fewer aches and pains.

But, as you'll read in this chapter, if you go on the EOD Diet *and* exercise, the strong medicine becomes stronger. Exercise is a uniquely powerful way to prevent disease and improve health. Among its many proven benefits, regular exercise can help you:

- Build muscle, shed fat, and control weight
- Boost energy and banish fatigue
- Brighten mood
- Clear up depression and anxiety
- Solve insomnia and other sleep problems
- Ease the impact of chronic stress
- Power up memory, concentration, and learning ability
- Prevent Alzheimer's disease
- Balance blood sugar, preventing or reversing prediabetes and type 2 diabetes
- Lower high blood pressure, a risk factor for heart attack and stroke
- Increase good (HDL) cholesterol, protecting your arteries
- Recover from a heart attack and prevent a second heart attack
- Prevent cancer and its recurrence
- Prevent osteoporosis
- Prevent osteoarthritis, and relieve knee or hip pain from osteoarthritis
- Prevent and relieve back pain

Research also shows exercise can help reduce the burden of a wide range of other diseases and health problems, like addiction, chronic fatigue syndrome, chronic heart failure, COPD (chronic obstructive pulmonary disease), fibromyalgia, intermittent claudication (leg cramps and pain from poor circulation), irregular heartbeat (atrial fibrillation), menopausal problems, multiple sclerosis, neck and shoulder pain, Parkinson's disease, prostate problems, and schizophrenia. And that's far from a complete list.

Bottom line: Exercise itself is powerful medicine for your body and mind. Combine it with the Every-Other-Day Diet, and you have an extra-strength approach to better health.

EOD Dieting and Exercise: Better Together

As a scientist devoted to dealing with the twin epidemics of obesity and heart disease, I'm well aware of the health-enhancing powers of exercise, so I decided to conduct studies to see what would happen when people went on the Every-Other-Day Diet and exercised a couple of days per week.[1]

I'd already discovered that EOD dieters *could* exercise, a scientific finding that really surprised me. I thought that EOD dieters would feel tired on Diet Day and avoid physical activity and exercise. But in a study of 16 people, published in *Nutrition Journal* in 2010, I found that folks didn't slow down on Diet Day. Once I discovered that people didn't retreat to the couch on Diet Day, I conducted another study on EOD dieting and exercise, trying to answer the following questions:

- Would a combination of the Every-Other-Day Diet and exercise trigger even more weight loss than EOD dieting alone?
- Would exercise make the EOD Diet even healthier for your heart?

- When was the best time of day to exercise on Diet Day, for maximum energy and minimum hunger? I didn't want people to be so hungry after exercising on Diet Day that they'd cheat on the diet.

The study involved 64 obese people (people who were 30 or more pounds overweight) and lasted eight weeks. The participants were divided into four groups:

- *People doing EOD dieting and exercise.* For their exercise, the study participants worked out on either a stationary bike or an elliptical machine, which combines leg and arm movements. They started with workouts of 25 minutes, building up to 40 minutes by the end of the study. They also gradually increased exercise intensity, which we measured using a heart rate monitor.
- *People doing only EOD dieting.*
- *People doing only exercise.*
- *People doing neither dieting nor exercise* (the control group).

My findings were remarkable: **People doing diet and exercise had twice as much weight loss as people doing only EOD dieting and not exercising.** The folks who just dieted lost an average of 6.6 pounds over the eight weeks of the study. But the folks who dieted and exercised lost *twice* as much weight, an average of 13.2 pounds. The people who exercised without dieting lost 2.2 pounds. The control group didn't lose any weight. An important point to note about the exercise-only group: It's *very* difficult to lose weight with exercise alone. Just do the math. Starting today, you can reduce your food intake by 1,000 calories and shed weight as your body burns stored fat for energy. But it would take several hours of walking to burn those same 1,000 calories!

Exercise is a powerful *addition* to EOD dieting, as you're learning in this chapter. And if you exercise while on the EOD Diet, you're also much more likely to *maintain* weight loss, for reasons we'll explain in a second—and permanent weight loss is the best result of any diet.

Diet and exercise resulted in participants' having more calorie-burning muscle. When most dieters lose weight, they lose body fat *and* muscle: 75% fat and 25% muscle. That's unfortunate, because losing muscle during dieting is a setup for weight *regain*. Here's what happens: Muscle is metabolically active—pound for pound, it burns *seven times* more calories than fat. So when a dieter has lost muscle during her diet, she burns fewer calories per day after the diet and slowly but surely gains back the weight she lost. That's the sad fate of 9 out of 10 dieters.

However, the group combining EOD dieting and exercise didn't lose *any* muscle during the eight weeks of the study—they lost only fat!

As I said a moment ago, that is a remarkable result, and it's probably one of the key factors that explains a major scientific finding I report at length in chapter 7, "The Every-Other-Day Success Program": EOD dieters *don't* regain their weight, compared to conventional dieters. Yes, the Every-Other-Day Diet is the first and only diet scientifically shown to help you not only lose weight—but also keep it off. You read that claim all the time, of course. But it's usually hope and hype. With the EOD Diet, it's *true.*

People who dieted and exercised banished more belly fat. The folks who were exercising and dieting lost an average of 3 inches from their waistlines. Those on the EOD Diet alone lost 2 inches. The exercisers who did not diet lost 1.2 inches.

The EOD Diet + exercise group had higher HDL levels. The EOD Diet + exercise group had the healthiest hearts, too. The exercise-and-diet combination produced a robust 12% drop in bad, artery-clogging LDL—and a whopping 18% increase in good, artery-clearing HDL. That's a very unique benefit. EOD dieting can lower LDL, and exercise can boost HDL, but only *combining them* does both.

Summing up: The combination of the Every-Other-Day Diet and exercise "produces superior changes in body weight, body composition and lipid [fat] indicators of heart disease risk" when compared with EOD dieting or exercise alone, I wrote in the journal *Obesity* in 2013. Or, in nonscientific lingo: if you want the best results, go on the Every-Other-Day Diet *and* exercise.

STEVE'S STORY: "I DON'T STOP EXERCISING ON DIET DAY."

Weight loss: 22 pounds

"I run for two miles, a couple of days a week," says Steve W., a 39-year-old sales director for a wireless phone company in Chicago, Illinois, and a former college football player who had seen his postcollege weight creep up slowly, from 185 to 228 pounds.

On the Every-Other-Day Diet *and* exercise, he lost 22 pounds in 12 weeks, and he is looking forward to losing a lot more.

"I've always been a fairly active fellow," he told us. "But now that I've lost all that weight, I have more energy, my back and ankles don't hurt when I run, and my cholesterol, blood pressure, and blood sugar levels are down.

"I don't stop exercising on Diet Day," he continued. "I run in the morning, drink a lot of water, and I'm fine until lunch. I don't feel any ill effects whatsoever."

The study described above showed what's happening to people's *bodies* on the EOD Diet. But what was happening in the *gym*? How did it feel to exercise on Diet Day? Did 500 calories fuel and support a workout, or were the EOD dieters weary, hungry, and unhappy? My study answered those questions, too.

It was easy to exercise on Diet Day. The folks in the study chose which day they'd exercise—Diet Day or Feast Day—and they chose both. In other words, people didn't have any problem exercising on Diet Day.

People didn't overeat when they exercised. When the folks in the study exercised in the *morning* on Diet Day, they were usually fine. They had a small snack midmorning, ate lunch, and didn't feel out of sorts; they cheated on the diet only about 10% of the time. (Hey, nobody's perfect.)

There are three best times to exercise on Diet Day.

Exercising in the afternoon wasn't the best strategy. Some participants reported being really hungry about 40 minutes after exercising if they exercised in the afternoon, and they cheated on the diet about 17% of the time, often eating both lunch *and* dinner and exceeding their 500 calories. Cheating 17% of the time isn't all that bad, in terms of sticking with the EOD Diet and losing weight. But it's not ideal. From that finding, we deduced that there are three ideal times to exercise on Diet Day:

1. *first thing in the morning*, eating your 100-calorie snack right afterward;
2. *right before lunch*; or
3. *right before dinner*, if you choose dinner as your Diet Day meal

Exercise boosts willpower and decreases bingeing and emotional eating. We also found that people who dieted *and* exercised were better able to say no to extra food on Diet Day, had less tendency to overeat in response to negative emotions, and binged less.

Bottom line: My studies show that the way to lose the *most* weight, retain the *most* calorie-burning muscle, trim the *most* belly fat, lower LDL *and* boost HDL cholesterol levels for an optimally healthy heart, and minimize self-destructive eating behaviors is by going on the Every-Other-Day Diet *and* getting regular exercise.

I want to repeat this fact—drive it home, really—because it's so important to your health and well-being: if you go on the EOD Diet *and* exercise, you will get the most benefits.

That's why I'm devoting the rest of this chapter to helping you exercise regularly.

ARE YOU A "REGULAR" EXERCISER?

What *is* "regular exercise," exactly? There are a lot of definitions out there, from the Centers for Disease Control and Prevention (CDC); from the US Department of Agriculture; from the Department of Health and Human Services; from the President's Council on Fitness, Sports & Nutrition; and from many other national organizations and associations. The CDC's guidelines for aerobic exercise are pretty typical:

1. *a minimum of 150 minutes a week of moderate-intensity exercise*: for example, 30 minutes of brisk walking, five days a week; or
2. *a minimum of 75 minutes a week of vigorous-intensity exercise (like jogging)*: for example, 25 minutes of jogging, three days a week.

Unfortunately, very few of us are guided by those guidelines. A survey by the American Heart Association found that 80% of us—4 out of 5—*don't* exercise regularly. So the obvious question is: If you're among the 80% of nonexercisers out there—if you're sedentary now, and need to form the exercise habit—what is the exercise you're most likely to *do*, a couple of days a week, week after week? Fortunately, there's a science-proven, low-tech, easy-does-it answer to that question: walking.

The National Weight Control Registry is a database of

lifestyle information about thousands of people who have lost at least 30 pounds and kept them off for at least one year. On average, those in the Registry have lost 66 pounds and have kept them off for 5.5 years. Among the many strategies used to lose weight and keep it off, 94% of people in the Registry increased their level of physical activity, and most of them did so by *walking*. My coauthor Bill was told this by James Hill, PhD, one of the founders of the Registry, a professor at the University of Colorado Health Sciences Center and director of the Center of Human Nutrition at the National Institutes of Health.

Walking is, of course, made up of *steps*. And many studies show the more steps you take, the less you weigh. The America On the Move study showed the average American takes only 5,117 steps per day—and the fewer steps a person takes, the higher is his or her body mass index (BMI), a standard measurement of body fat.[2] A BMI of 25 to 29.9 is categorized as overweight; 30 and above is called obese. (Details of how to measure BMI are given in chapter 1.) In the study, people who were obese walked an average of 1,500 fewer steps than people who were overweight or normal weight.

In another study, from the Center for Physical Activity and Health at the University of Tennessee, people who walked an average of 10,023 steps a day had an average BMI of 24.1— normal weight—while people who took fewer than 10,000 steps were either overweight or obese.[3]

And in a study from the Prevention Research Center at the University of South Carolina, people with an average of 9,000 or more steps per day were more likely to be normal weight, and people with fewer than 5,000 steps were more likely to be obese.[4]

If you don't exercise regularly now, walking is a great way to start—and in this chapter you'll find a pedometer-based walking program that we feel is the ideal way to start and maintain an exercise routine, particularly for folks who need to lose weight. But if walking isn't for you, don't worry. The key to regular exercise, say experts, is to find a physical activity that you *enjoy*—because that's the activity you'll do regularly. Maybe it's gardening, dancing, or swimming; or maybe it's a combination of different activities, which helps keep you from becoming bored.

If you're already exercising regularly, we have tips for you, too, from a leading researcher in exercise psychology who has figured out why people typically stop exercising (lack of willpower) and exactly what to do about it. Let's take a look at that researcher's ideas.

FIVE SECRETS OF REGULAR EXERCISE

Is your garage or basement the Museum of Good Intentions, with dusty displays of a NordicTrack, Bowflex, or other exercise machines you ordered with enthusiasm but used only for a few weeks or months? If so, you're far from alone. There are a lot of resolutions that fail because of lack of resolve or willpower, and exercising regularly is certainly one of them. Half of all people who start an exercise routine stop within six months.

But there are several strategies to make sure you *always* have enough willpower to exercise, no matter what type of exercise you choose, says Kathleen Martin Ginis, PhD, a professor of health and exercise psychology in the Department of Kinesiology at McMaster University in Canada.

The surprising fact is that willpower is *not* an unlimited resource, and that you have to manage and conserve it, so there's always enough when you need it.

"Willpower can weaken and then fatigue completely—just like a muscle you're using to lift weights," Dr. Martin Ginis explained. "This 'limited strength model of willpower'—first described by Roy Baumeister, PhD, at Florida State—says that willpower is a *finite, renewable* resource that is drained when you try to control your behaviors, thoughts or emotions." At that point, you have to *wait* for willpower to "recover" before you can use it again, she said. And knowing how to keep the "power" in "willpower" can make all the difference in whether or not you exercise regularly.

Below are Dr. Martin Ginis's suggestions for always having plenty of willpower to get out and exercise.

1. Make a plan

"This is a particularly important for people starting an exercise program," she said. "You have to think through where you're going to exercise, what exercise you'll do when you get there, how you'll fit the exercise into your day, and what you'll do if and when the exercise starts to feel uncomfortable.

"Because there's so much thinking and planning around exercise—all of which demand willpower—the best strategy is to plan your exercise in advance.

"For example, at the beginning of the month, or the beginning of the week, take out a calendar and figure out the days you'll be exercising, and the time of day you'll do it.

"This type of advance planning removes the need for a lot

of daily self-control. When the planned time for exercise rolls around, you don't have to use your limited willpower making a decision whether or not to exercise—the decision is already made. Just get up out of your chair and go.

"Planning is an astoundingly effective strategy for not draining willpower—and for maintaining regular exercise," she said.

2. Exercise in the morning

This is an effective strategy for those who are morning people. "You exercise before other activities drain willpower," Dr. Martin Ginis said.

3. Take a break and then exercise

"Rest is always the best way to replenish willpower," she said. "Take 10 to 15 minutes, close your eyes, and meditate or catnap. Then go out and exercise."

4. Boost your mood

"A good mood helps you muster up willpower," she said. "Listen to music you like. Read a joke book."

5. Strengthen your willpower by using it

"If you consistently use your willpower—resisting a second piece of chocolate cake, stopping yourself from checking your email every 15 minutes, resisting the urge to hit the snooze button when your alarm goes off in the morning—you'll gradually increase the strength of your willpower, so that it more readily responds when you need it for any activity," she said.

"Willpower is like a muscle," she emphasized. "Using it is temporarily draining, but builds greater strength for the next time you want to 'exercise' self-control."

Behavioral scientists say there are three more essential strategies to making a positive change in your life, such as forming and maintaining an exercise habit:

1. Set a goal.
2. Monitor yourself.
3. Relish the satisfaction of success once you reach your goal.

There's a simple device you can buy for a few bucks that allows you to do those three very things: a pedometer.

YOUR PEDOMETER-BASED WALKING PROGRAM

A *pedometer* is a small device you clip to your belt or waistband or carry in your pocket, where it counts and displays the number of steps you take each day. Using a pedometer is like having access to a coach who is *always* helping you maintain or increase your level of physical activity. When researchers from Stanford analyzed 26 studies on pedometers and walking, involving nearly 3,000 people, they found that those using a pedometer increased their daily activity by an average of nearly 2,500 steps per day—a little more than one mile.[5] If you're not already a regular exerciser, a pedometer-based walking program is a great way to get started. Here's how to choose a pedometer and get going.

THE PRIMO PEDOMETER

Ready to put on a pedometer and see where it takes you? You'll quickly discover there are *hundreds* of pedometers on the market. How do you choose? Do what we did: ask a world-class pedometer expert.

"I recommend the Omron HJ-112, which is *very* reliable," Bill was told by Caroline Richardson, MD, one of the world's leading experts in using pedometers for weight control and wellness, an associate professor in the Department of Family Medicine at the University of Michigan, and a researcher at the Ann Arbor Veterans Administration Center for Clinical Management Research. "It's accurate, durable, easy to use, and cheap." (You can find one on amazon.com for $22.99, along with nearly 3,000 5-star reviews.)

You can put this pedometer in your pocket or in your pocketbook, or clip it to your belt or waistband—it's accurate in *any* position. That's not the case with many other pedometers, which have to be vertical to register a step. And accuracy is crucial: you don't want a pedometer that undercounts (so you never reach your goal) or overcounts (so you think you've reached it but you haven't).

A slightly more expensive Omron pedometer—the HJ720-ITC—has a USB port, so you can upload your steps into accompanying software that helps you track (and reach) your goals; this is the pedometer Dr. Richardson uses in all her studies on pedometers and health.

Some pedometers—like the wireless Fitbit—automatically upload your step info to a computer program or smartphone

(continued)

application that tracks steps. And Fitbit (and several other wireless pedometers) are compatible with the smartphone programs from www.myfitnesspal.com, which are used by hundreds of thousands of people to keep track of daily calories.

Although the Omron models are her favorites, there are many other good devices available, Dr. Richardson said. "There are hundreds of new pedometers every year, with prices dropping and the quality increasing—everybody can find a pedometer that works for them."

Figure Out Your Daily Step Count

You've bought your pedometer and are ready to increase your steps. Don't do it—at least not for the first week. "Wear a pedometer for seven days to determine your baseline," said Caroline Richardson, MD, one of the world's leading experts in using pedometers for weight control and wellness, an associate professor in the Department of Family Medicine at the University of Michigan, and a researcher at the Ann Arbor Veterans Administration Center for Clinical Management Research. Here's her step-by-step method for determining your daily average of steps, or baseline:

1. Each night at bedtime, write down your steps for that day.
2. After seven days, add up the week's total of steps. (Some pedometers, like the Omron HJ-112, keep a daily record of the previous seven days of steps.)
3. Divide the number by 7 to get your daily average.

That's your baseline—and now you're ready to increase it! Add 1,200 steps per day for the first week: if your baseline was 5,000, your goal is to walk 6,200 steps per day. "That's enough steps to be a bit challenging, but not so many that it's impossible," Dr. Richardson said.

Then add an additional 1,200 the second week (so you are at 7,400 steps per day); and 1,200 more the third week (so you're at 8,200 per day); and so on, until you've reached 10,000 steps per day. However, Dr. Richardson also advised *individualizing* those increases, depending on your situation. For example, if you're obese or have a chronic disease, consider increasing your baseline by only 600 to 800 steps per day for the first week. If your baseline was 5,000, your goal is to walk 5,600 steps per day the first week; 6,200 steps per day the second week; and so on.

"With my patients, I constantly adjust the 1,200-per-day [step] number and overall number, depending on what the person can do," she said. "If he's not making his goal, or only half his goal, I don't add 1,200 steps per week."

How do you increase your steps week by week? The obvious way is to go for a daily walk of 30 minutes or more. Walking briskly, you can log 3,000 steps in about 30 minutes. Several shorter walks—of 5, 10, or 15 minutes—are also a good strategy.

What's important is that you actually *take* those steps. When researchers in the Department of Sports Medicine at the University of Southern Maine studied 34 people involved in an eight-week "pedometer-based lifestyle intervention," they found the walkers typically chose one or more of 10 basic strategies to increase their daily steps.[6]

They walked

- before work
- to a meeting or on a work-related errand
- using the stairs, rather than the elevator
- at lunch
- after work
- to a destination like work or a store
- after parking farther away from a destination than usual
- with the dog
- on the weekend
- while traveling

My preference: walking to work. I take the train to and from work every day. Going to work, I get off at a station two miles away from the University of Illinois and walk the rest of the way. Coming home, I walk two miles to that same station. That's 8,000 steps worth of walking, so I know I'm meeting the 10,000-step goal every day.

Bill wears a pedometer from when he gets up in the morning to when he goes to bed at night. On at least four days a week, he logs 4,000 to 6,000 steps per day by going on a walk of 45 to 60 minutes.

STEP UP TO FITNESS—MORE IDEAS FOR GETTING EXTRA STEPS

James Hill, PhD, a professor at the University of Colorado Health Sciences Center, has plenty of ideas for how to build more steps into your day:

At work

- Take two 10-minute walks during the day.
- Walk to a restroom, soda machine, or copy machine on a different floor.
- Walk a few laps around your floor during breaks.
- Take 5-minute walking breaks from your computer.
- Get off the bus earlier before work and walk the extra blocks to work.
- Walk around while using a speakerphone, cordless phone, or mobile phone.
- Find a lunch spot that is at least a 10-minute walk each way to/from your office.

Out and about

- Return your grocery cart to the designated storage area.
- Walk around the airport while waiting for your plane.
- Make several trips to unload your groceries from your car.
- Avoid the drive-thru—get out of your car and walk inside.
- Walk around the local mall.
- Walk to your nearest mailbox to mail a letter, instead of leaving it for the mail carrier to pick up.
- Walk around the field or gym at your kids' games.
- Pick up litter in your neighborhood or park.

At home with family and friends

- Walk around the living room during TV commercials. There's scientific proof for this idea. In a recent

(continued)

study conducted by researchers at the National Cancer Institute, sedentary, overweight people did "TV Commercial Stepping" during 90 minutes of daily TV watching.[7] After six months, their average daily step count had increased from 4,611 to 7,605. A similar group assigned to daily walking with a pedometer increased their steps from 4,909 to 7,865. In other words, *both* strategies worked to increase steps.

- Go up and down the stairs with laundry or other household items separately, instead of combining trips.
- Empty wastebaskets every day.
- Walk to a neighbor's or friend's house instead of phoning.

Make the Small Changes That Drive Success

If you've never exercised before, it's unrealistic to think that you're going to instantly be a marathoner. The trick is to set realistic, achievable goals and to increase your activity in small amounts.

"Small changes drive success," Dr. Hill said. He didn't always think that way. But now he knows better.

"I spent most of my career trying to get people to make *big* lifestyle changes," he said. "They made them—but they didn't stick with them. I've done a total about-face in my approach to lifestyle change because now I understand that *small changes* are what work."

How does a pedometer fit into that philosophy?

"Let me give you an example," Dr. Hill said. "A patient of mine decides to follow the physical activity recommendations to get anywhere from 30 to 90 minutes of moderate to intense physical activity on most days of the week. Well, if he's like many of the overweight people I work with, he probably hasn't been off the couch in six months. Even 30 minutes of physical activity isn't going to be easy for him. But he's determined to give it a try. He joins a gym, works out a couple of days a week for two to three weeks—and then stops. *Why* did he stop? Because the change was too big to sustain.

"But with a pedometer, he doesn't have to achieve a big goal right away, like exercising for 30 minutes most days of the week. Instead, he determines how many steps he takes each day, and then he increases the number by a *little bit*. He moves *toward* his goal, little by little."

Small changes allow you to get motivated and stay motivated "until you've made a big, extraordinary change," Dr. Hill said. And when you've achieved a big change, through a series of small changes, it's much more likely you'll *stay* changed.

It's also important to set a goal for yourself—for example, getting to 10,000 steps in a pedometer program. Whatever your pace in reaching the 10,000-steps-per-day level, Dr. Richardson thinks that number of daily steps is a good goal for most people—*because* it's not easy to achieve. "It's a challenge to reach 10,000 steps," she said. "You have to take a 60-minute walk per day, or a lot of little walks throughout the day. And a challenge is *good*.

"Thousands of studies on goal setting show that *high, hard goals* are what maximize success—and it doesn't matter how high and hard they are, as long as the person thinks there is a reasonable chance of achieving the goal. People *like* high, hard goals—they're motivating and fun."

Believe in Yourself

Another important part of increasing your level of physical activity is what behavioral scientists call *self-efficacy*, says Dr. Richardson. You have to *believe* you can reach the goal. With a pedometer, that's easy. She gives an example:

"I tell one of my patients to increase her steps by 1,000 a day. She walks down the hall and back and sees that she's just put 100 steps on her pedometer. She says to herself, 'Wow, I just got 100 steps—I'm going to walk down that hall again.'"

That feel-good experience is quite different from what typically happens when a well-meaning doctor tells you to "get more exercise."

"When you're sedentary and a physician tells you to exercise more, you really don't know where to start," Dr. Richardson said. You might work out too hard and feel lousy afterward. And you might still feel like a failure, because you really don't know if you exercised enough. But with a pedometer, you have a concrete goal. You know exactly what you need to do and whether you've done it or not. And when you do it, you feel good about yourself.

So whether you decide to walk using a pedometer, or jog a couple of days a week, or ride a stationary bicycle, or you choose another type of physical activity, try to find a way to go on the Every-Other-Day Diet *and* exercise regularly. You'll lose more weight, trim more belly fat, and your heart will be that much healthier. Your body was built to move. If you're not exercising regularly now, it might be a bit hard to get moving at first. But once you do, you'll be glad you did!

EOD—EASY AS 1-2-3

1. Appreciate the unique pound-shedding power of combining the EOD Diet with regular exercise.
2. Use the Five Secrets of Regular Exercise to start an exercise program and stay on track.
3. Walk. It's the most popular form of exercise among people who successfully lose weight. Use a pedometer to help you walk regularly.

The Every-Other-Day Success Program: The Science-Proven Way to Keep the Weight Off

Five out of six dieters regain their weight; you won't be one of them

You've probably heard the famous Mark Twain quote about quitting smoking. "It's easy," he said. "I've done it hundreds of times." Many of us could say something very similar about losing weight, and that probably includes you. If you're reading this book, it's likely you've read other diet books, tried their diets, lost weight, and then gained the weight back—every single pound, every single time. Welcome to the club, which has about 100 million members.

A recent national survey found that 55% of American adults are currently on a weight-loss diet. But research also shows that 5 out of 6 people who diet and lose weight subsequently *regain* their weight—*all* of it, after just one year. That's right: for every 6 people who go on a diet and lose weight, only 1 is trimmer a year later. And scientists now understand why.

THE REASONS YOU REGAIN THE WEIGHT

When you lose a lot of weight, your body's metabolism—the pace at which it burns calories—resets itself. Moment by moment, day by day, *you burn fewer calories than you did before you lost weight.*

Scientists call this phenomena *adaptive thermogenesis.* They don't know exactly why it happens. But they do have an evolutionary theory, which could be called the Survival of the Fattest. It posits that the body has a mind of its own; when you dieted, it thought its food supply was threatened. Now it thinks it has to preserve fat for you to stay alive. So your body has decided to burn fewer calories—for the rest of your life, which it hopes is as long as possible.

Say, for example, that you weighed 250 pounds, lost 50, and now weigh 200 pounds. If you compare your daily caloric needs to an adult who has *always* weighed 200 pounds—an adult who has never dieted—you, the ex-dieter, need to eat 15% to 25% *fewer* calories to maintain the same weight of 200 pounds. That's because the calories the ex-dieter takes in are burned much more slowly than the calories the "always-200-pounder" ingests.

A moderately active man who has trimmed down to

200 pounds has a daily maintenance level of about 3,250 calories. But postdiet, he needs to eat only about 2,500 calories
to maintain his weight, or *750 calories less per day* than a
similarly active man who has always weighed 200 pounds.
That's nearly an entire meal less, every day!

Forgoing an entire meal every day is no picnic—literally!
Five out of six of us can't do it. And 5 out of 6 of us regain the
weight.

There's a second reason why weight regain is so common.
During traditional dieting, you shed metabolically active,
calorie-burning *muscle* along with fat, which further inter-
feres with your ability to burn up rather than store postdiet
calories. And if you regain weight, you're likely to regain most
of it as *fat*, which is why many dieters don't just return to
their old weight; with less muscle to burn calories, they end
up heavier than ever.

Another reason you regain weight: Your body doesn't only
reset its metabolism after a significant weight loss to protect
you from starvation. It's a lot smarter than that. It also starts to
pump out a different ratio of the hormones that control your
appetite. You manufacture more *ghrelin*, the hormone that
increases hunger. You manufacture less *leptin*, the hormone
that *decreases* hunger. In short, you're hungrier. And you eat
more.

THE EVERY-OTHER-DAY SUCCESS PROGRAM: REVERSING THE REASONS FOR REGAIN

So your metabolism has slowed to a crawl, forcing you to eat
about one-third less than a nondieter to maintain the same

weight. There's a hunger hormone sitting on your shoulder like a devil, whispering, *Eat, eat, eat.* And to make matters worse, a bunch of your muscle has abandoned ship. What's a dieter to do?

Well, other diet books either ignore this rebound effect or mislead the reader about it, assuring dieters they won't regain their weight—with no scientific evidence to support the claim.

The Every-Other-Day Diet is different. I don't avoid or whitewash this issue. Instead, I offer the Every-Other-Day Success Program—a new, every-other-day pattern of eating, similar to the diet itself, but not as low in calories. Once you reach your goal weight, you start the EOD Success Program. And like the Every-Other-Day Diet, the Success Program is supported by scientific research—my *newest* research, which shows that people who lose weight on the EOD Diet and then go on the Success Program *don't* regain that weight. Before we get to those spectacular results, I'm sure you're wondering just how the Success Program works.

WHAT IS THE EVERY-OTHER-DAY SUCCESS PROGRAM?

You transition to the EOD Success Program as soon as you reach your goal weight. And the essence of the program couldn't be simpler:

> *Eat 1,000 calories on Monday, Wednesday, and Friday (Success Days), and eat as much as you want,*

and whatever you want, on the other days of the week (Feast Days).

My study participants were asked to limit their calories every other day, and they did—but only during the week! Most of them decided to take the weekend off. And that turned out just fine. They still maintained their weight loss and all the other healthful changes they had achieved while on the EOD Diet. (And that was okay with me. As a scientist, I'm most interested in what *really* works, not an approach I think *might* work.)

During the EOD Diet, Diet Day typically consisted of one 400-calorie meal and one 100-calorie snack. During the EOD Success Program, Success Day consists of two 400-calorie meals and two 100-calorie snacks. You can consume those meals and snacks in any pattern of daily eating that you prefer—one large meal, three smaller meals—as long as you don't exceed 1,000 calories.

Feast Days are the same as they were on the EOD Diet: eat all the food you want, and eat any food you want. However, because this is a lifelong program, my study participants were counseled about healthy food choices and lifestyle habits to support a lifetime of weight maintenance and good health. You'll find similar information later in this chapter. But before getting to that practical info, let's take a closer look at the results of my study on the Success Program—results that will give you the confidence you need to embark on this lifelong journey to weight maintenance.

SPECTACULAR RESULTS IN WEIGHT LOSS *AND* IN WEIGHT MAINTENANCE

In chapter 1, I describe the results of many of the studies I've conducted on the Every-Other-Day Diet, including the results from the first year of an ongoing three-year study sponsored by the National Institutes of Health (NIH). But the NIH study is unique. It doesn't just look at the Every-Other-Day Diet. It also looks at the Every-Other-Day Success Program.

This three-year study consists of three one-year experiments. For the first six months of the year, the participants are on the EOD Diet, *losing* weight. For the next six months they are on the Every-Other-Day Success Program, *maintaining* weight.

I'm delighted to report (as I did in November 2013, at the annual "ObesityWeek" conference, the world's most prestigious conference on obesity and weight loss[1]) that *both* every-other-day programs work: on the Every-Other-Day Diet people shed pounds; and on the Every-Other-Day Success Program people maintain that weight loss. Let's take a closer look at those results—and what they mean for *you*.

You'll eat fewer calories automatically. The Every-Other-Day Success Program was originally designed to provide 50% of normal calories on one day (Success Day) and 150% of normal calories on the next (Feast Day). My first surprise: hardly anybody could eat 150% of their Feast Day calories in a single day! The study participants topped out at an average of 125%.

In other words, whatever metabolic and hormonal forces were in play, the unique effect of EOD eating stopped those former dieters from overeating. They *automatically* ate the more limited amount of calories necessary for weight maintenance!

You'll keep losing weight—and keep it off. If you're sitting down, stand up and cheer! Because the study results are worth celebrating.

While on the EOD Diet, the participants in the study lost from 15 to 50 pounds, with an average loss of 25 pounds. While on the EOD Success Program, those same dieters gained back an average of 1 pound. (That's right—*1 pound*.)

Bottom line: Participants hardly regained any weight. They maintained their weight loss. Where 5 out of 6 dieters on other diets failed, they succeeded. And they did that by continuing the EOD pattern: eating 1,000 calories one day and all they wanted the next.

You'll lose fat, not muscle. As I pointed out previously, people lose 75% fat and 25% muscle on a typical diet, and shedding all that muscle sabotages the ability to maintain weight loss. In this study, as in all of my previous studies on the Every-Other-Day Diet, the participants shed most of their weight as fat, and very little as muscle.

The average weight loss was 25 pounds:

- 23 pounds of that was fat;
- 2 pounds was muscle

That's a big reason why the Every-Other-Day Success Program *is* a success.

You'll bust belly fat, big-time. The EOD Diet whittled

away the waistlines of the study participants, with an average decrease of more than 5 inches. (The men lost more belly fat than the women, because they had more to begin with.) And that extra abdominal fat wasn't regained on the Success Program:

- Belly fat lost on the EOD Diet: 2 to 6 pounds
- Belly fat regained on the EOD Success Program: 0 pounds
- Average waistline reduced on the EOD Diet: 5½ inches
- Average waistline regained on the EOD Success Program: 0 inches

Trimming tummy fat does more than boost your self-esteem and help you get back into your skinny jeans. A bulging belly is the outward sign of excess *visceral* fat, the "deep" fat that wraps around your inner organs and ruins your health. Every extra pound of visceral fat translates into higher risk for heart disease, stroke, and type 2 diabetes. Likewise, every pound you lose lowers your risk.

You'll continue to protect your heart. In my NIH study, participants lowered their LDL cholesterol by an average of 11% during the diet, and that decrease continued during the Success Program. They lowered their blood pressure by an average of 9 points, and that drop continued during the Success Program. They decreased their fasting glucose by 8% (high glucose is a risk factor for both heart disease and type 2 diabetes), and that decrease continued during the Success Program.

As you can see, both the Every-Other-Day Diet and the Every-Other-Day Success Program *work.*

- You lose weight and don't regain it.
- You lose fat (but not muscle), and the fat stays away.
- You trim inches off your waistline, and they don't inch back.
- LDL cholesterol drops and stays down
- Blood pressure lowers and stays lower.
- Glucose levels fall and don't go back up.

VICTORIA'S STORY: "IT WILL BE EASY TO CONTROL MY WEIGHT FOR THE REST OF MY LIFE."

Weight loss: 27 pounds

A medical technician and Chicago resident, 33-year-old, 5'5" Victoria weighed 245 pounds, until she went on the Every-Other-Day Diet.

"I have two school-age children and a full-time job, and I'm very busy, without much time to cook," she said. "Before going on the diet, I ate whatever I wanted to—fast foods, fried foods, just grabbing something on the go."

The Every-Other-Day Diet helped her slow down a bit and plan a lot of meals for both herself and her kids, both on Diet Day and on Feast Day, and she slowly but surely began to shed pounds, hitting 218 pounds.

When we talked with her, she had been on the Every-Other-Day Success Program for a few months and had lost 27 pounds. "I'm *still* losing 1 to 2 pounds per week, compared to the 2 or 3 pounds per week while I was on the diet," she said. "I just mimic what I did on the diet."

(continued)

On Success Day, she controls her hunger by drinking tea and chewing gum. She also enjoys eating the same frozen foods she ate on Diet Day, because they taste good and are convenient, but now she can have two entrées instead of one.

On Feast Day, Victoria has started to eat more fresh food, such as salads, steamed vegetables, and fruit. And she's exercising regularly, working out two or three times a week.

Victoria is very intent on success because she's dieted before, lost the weight, and has *always* regained it.

"Success Day is very important to me because I want to keep the weight off," she said. "With other diets, they lasted a few months, and that's it. With the Every-Other-Day Success Program, it will be easy to control my weight for the rest of my life—and that's what I'm going to do!"

KEEP UP THE GOOD WORK!

There are a lot of habits I recommended that you start while on the EOD Diet, to help you maximize weight loss and good health, and I hope you keep on doing them! We'll review them below.

Get regular exercise. In chapter 6, I discussed the power of combining the Every-Other-Day Diet with regular exercise and introduced you to a pedometer-based walking program. If you started walking (or doing any other type of regular exercise) while on the EOD Diet, congratulations—don't stop now! Here's why. A national registry of thousands of people who have lost weight and kept it off for at least one year shows that 94% of them increased their physical activity level. Most of them did so by walking.

And when researchers at Harvard Medical School studied more than 4,500 women age 26 to 45 who had lost weight, they found that those who added just 30 minutes of physical activity to their daily routine (brisk walking was a favorite) were 52% less likely to regain a lot of weight in the two years after they shed the pounds.[2]

If you haven't read chapter 6—"Every-Other-Day Dieting and Exercise"—I strongly encourage you to do so. And I also strongly encourage you to do what that chapter says to do: exercise regularly, using either the pedometer-based walking program described in the chapter or some other form of exercise.

Weigh yourself every day. Studies show this habit not only helps with weight loss, but also with weight maintenance, as we discussed earlier. If, for whatever reason, you see the pounds creeping back on, go back on the EOD Diet until you've returned to your goal weight—and then restart the Success Program.

Drink plenty of water. Drinking an 8-ounce glass of water 15 or 30 minutes before each meal is a great way to control hunger and calorie intake on Success Day, as we discussed earlier. Drinking water throughout the day also helps.

Chew gum. This is another simple habit that can improve your chances of long-term weight maintenance. It cuts hunger and appetite and increases alertness. It even burns a few extra calories.

CALORIE COUNTING MADE EASY

There are a lot of different ways to take in the 1,000 calories of Success Day—one, two, or three meals, and one or two snacks. Any combination works, as long as you don't exceed the calorie limit. What's the best way to keep track of those calories? Let me count the ways you can count the calories.

Use chapters 4 and 5. You can prepare the calorie-controlled recipes and snacks from chapter 4: one 400-calorie lunch, one 400-calorie dinner, and two 100-calorie snacks to total 1,000 calories. Or choose packaged meals and snacks from chapter 5 that add up to 1,000 calories.

Buy cookbooks featuring meals of 400 calories or less. For more recipes, you can also buy and use one or more of the many cookbooks that offer 400- and 500-calorie meals and 100-calorie snacks. Some of our favorites: *400 Calorie Fix Cookbook*; *EatingWell 500-Calorie Dinners*; *Mix & Match Low-Calorie Cookbook* from CookingLight (the breakfast and lunch recipes are under 400 calories, and the dinner recipes are under 500); *500 400-Calorie Recipes*; the 400 Calorie series from Good Housekeeping (which includes a general cookbook and cookbooks featuring chicken, Italian, vegetarian, and comfort foods); *The Complete Idiot's Guide to 200-300-400 Calorie Meals*; and *The 100-Calorie Snack Cookbook*.

Google "400-calorie recipes." You'll get more than three million hits!

Download a calorie-counting app or buy a calorie counter. Use a smartphone app for calorie counting, like MyFitnessPal or Lose It! Apps are particularly efficient for calorie counting: they're always with you and they're easy to use. You can also go the old-fashioned route and buy a book to help you with calorie counting. One of the most popular is *The CalorieKing Calorie, Fat, & Carbohydrate Counter 2013.*

Use the calorie cheat sheet (below) of food categories as a guide: An interesting and helpful way to think about calories is to think of foods in terms of *calories per pound,* advises Jeffrey Novick, MS, RD, a dietitian and nutritionist in California who has worked with Whole Foods in developing their Wellness Club. Of course, you wouldn't eat a pound of broccoli or a pound of butter. But a pound-for-pound comparison between the two foods shows just how many calories each packs and the differences between them—and why emphasizing vegetables, fresh fruits, whole grains, legumes, and lean proteins can help you stay within the 1,000-calorie limit of Success Day. Here is a list of some food categories and their calories per pound, in general:

- *Vegetables:* 100 to 200 calories per pound of food
- *Fresh fruits:* 200 to 300 calories per pound of food
- *Whole grains and legumes:* 500 calories per pound of food
- *Lean proteins, like seafood and the white meat of chicken:* 600 to 650 calories per pound of food

(continued)

- *Fattier proteins, like a steak served at a restaurant specializing in "premium" steaks:* 1,000 calories per pound of food
- *Refined, processed carbohydrates, such as breads, bagels, and crackers:* 1,200 to 1,500 calories per pound of food
- *Junk food, such as sugary cookies made with white flour:* 2,000 calories per pound of food
- *Nuts and seeds:* 2,800 calories per pound of food
- *Oils and fats:* 4,000 calories per pound of food

Not to worry: Calorie counting isn't forever. If you're like most people, you tend to eat the same one or two dozen foods over and over. After two to three months, you won't need any assistance in knowing how many calories you're taking in; it will be obvious to you.

MINDFUL EATING AND PORTION CONTROL: TWO OTHER KEYS TO WEIGHT MAINTENANCE

In addition to the tips we've already given you in this book, I want to discuss two others that will go a long way toward helping you maintain your weight loss.

Maintaining your weight loss isn't just about *what* you eat. It's also about *why* you eat. And what you do *when* you eat. Maybe there are times when you eat not because you feel *hungry*, but because you feel *lousy*. You use food to tranquilize negative emotions, ease stress, or relieve boredom.

Maybe there are food "cues" that you always respond to—see a cookie, eat a cookie—whether you're hungry or not.

And maybe there are times (maybe even most of the time) when you don't pay attention to the smell and taste and sensual enjoyment of eating. Instead, you eat in a rush—in the car or in front of the TV—barely noticing the food.

Research links these three habits—what scientists call *emotional eating, external eating,* and *distracted eating*—to overweight and obesity. But there's a habit that's pretty much the exact *opposite* of emotional, distracted, and external eating. And many studies, as I'll describe in a moment, link this habit to successful weight maintenance. It's called *mindful eating.*

Mindful eating is being aware of your emotions and moods in the moment—not judging them, not trying to get rid of them, just *observing* and *accepting* them—and therefore not letting anxiety, depression, boredom, or stress compel you to eat when you're not hungry.

Mindful eating is not letting old habits rule your life, but instead taking a step back—paying attention to your hunger and desires in the present moment—and deciding whether or not you *really* want those cookies. And even if you decide to eat cookies, maybe you decide to eat just one or two, and not the whole bag.

Mindful eating is paying attention to eating when you're eating. You notice the smell, taste, and texture of the food, and you eat slowly enough to *enjoy* it. You don't do anything else while you eat. Mindful eating is having an *intention*—maintaining your weight loss—and then having the *attention* to accomplish it.

I think mindful eating is one of the most powerful and important aids to success on the Every-Other-Day Success Program. The participants in my NIH-sponsored study were taught the skill. Plus, there's a lot of scientific research supporting the role of mindful eating in controlling weight. Some recent studies found the following:

If you're distracted, you eat more—a lot more. When a team of UK researchers analyzed studies on "eating attentively," they found that people who were distracted during eating ate a lot more food—up to 76% more than people who were attentive while eating. "Attentive eating is likely to influence food intake," wrote the researchers in the *American Journal of Clinical Nutrition*.[3]

If you eat mindfully, you eat smaller portions of high-calorie foods. In a study of 171 people published in the scientific journal *Appetite*, those who were more "mindful eaters" ate smaller portions of high-calorie foods.[4]

If you're mindful, you have fewer cravings and do less emotional eating. In a study by Dutch researchers, 26 women took a training course in mindful eating and as a result had fewer food cravings, and did less emotional and external eating. "Mindfulness practice can be an effective way to reduce...problematic eating behavior," wrote the researchers in *Appetite*.[5]

When you're mindful, **your brain *is less preoccupied with food!*** Researchers at Wake Forest University School of Medicine conducted brain scans (functional magnetic resonance imaging, or fMRI) on 19 obese people after they ate breakfast and weren't allowed to eat again for nearly three hours. Those with more mindfulness had "greater...efficiency" in their "brain networks," indicating they were less preoccupied with eating again.[6]

Mindfulness = weight maintenance. Researchers at the Osher Center for Integrative Medicine at the University of California, San Francisco, studied 47 overweight and obese women, dividing them into two groups. One group received mindfulness training aimed at reducing "stress eating" and one group didn't. After four months, the mindful group was less anxious, had less external-based eating, pumped out less of the stress hormone cortisol, and maintained their weight. Meanwhile, the nonmindful group gained weight.[7]

How to be a mindful eater

One of the top experts on mindful eating is Michelle May, MD, founder and CEO of the Am I Hungry? Mindful Eating Workshops, and author of *Eat What You Love, Love What You Eat* and several other books on mindful eating. Here are some of the key principles of mindful eating that Dr. May has shared with Bill. We'd like to note that Dr. May does not endorse the Every-Other-Day Diet, the Every-Other-Day Success Program, or any other weight-loss program or diet. But because her recommendations about mindful eating are uniquely insightful and effective, we wanted to share them with you.

Before you eat, ask yourself: "Why am I eating?" "People eat for reasons other than hunger," Dr. May said. "Often the cues are emotional, such as loneliness, depression, anxiety, stress, or boredom. These cues override our *internal* cues of hunger and fullness, and send you in the direction of comforting, convenient, and calorie-dense foods. And because you're not hungry when you *start* to eat, you don't know when to stop. You eat until the food is gone.

"Instead," she says, "ask yourself this simple question before you eat: 'Why am I eating?'

"Put a speed bump—a pause—between wanting to eat and starting to eat. Take a moment to realize what's really going on, whether you're physically hungry or responding to an emotional cue. If you discover you're not hungry, make a choice whether to use food to deal with something that isn't a physical need for food or to redirect your attention to something else until you're actually hungry."

Learn to recognize the physical signs of hunger. How can you tell whether or not you're hungry? *Scan* your body—particularly your stomach—for physical signs, Dr. May advises. "Get quiet for a moment," she said. "Scan your body from head to toe. Look for clues that your desire to eat isn't hunger, such as tension in your body, or pain, or worried thoughts. Also look for clues that your desire to eat *is* hunger, like a hollow or empty feeling in your stomach, or rumbling and growling. Do this scan whenever you feel like eating, and also about every three hours throughout the day, to see if you're truly hungry and need to eat."

Redirect your attention. If you're not hungry, one strategy is to distract yourself rather than eat, Dr. May said. Go for a walk. Pet your dog. Take a shower. Brush your teeth. Do your nails. Or, if you've identified the underlying emotional need that you're looking for food to satisfy, meet the need instead, in a small way. "Maybe you're overworked and stressed out and need a vacation," Dr. May said. "Take a few minutes to surf online and look at a travel site, or visualize being on vacation and resting in a hammock, or take a few deep breaths."

Learn to recognize when you feel full. Being able to decide not to eat when you're not hungry is one feature of mindful eating. Deciding to stop eating when you're comfortably full is another.

"Mindful eating is not about *being good* but about *feeling good*," said Dr. May. "Identify signs of fullness and stop when you feel comfortable. A smart idea for figuring out when you're full: set an intention before you eat. Ask yourself, 'How do I want to feel when I'm done?' You probably want to feel good, energetic, and satisfied, not bad, tired, and stuffed," Dr. May said.

PORTION SIZES: DON'T SUPERSIZE YOURSELF

There's another habit that's probably every bit as important as mindful eating: *controlling portion size.* In fact, many nutritional scientists think the trend toward ever-bigger portions— in supermarkets, restaurants, convenience stores, at home, and even in cookbooks—is *the* main reason why so many us have become overweight or obese. There's a lot of evidence supporting that perspective. For example, researchers in the Department of Nutrition at the University of North Carolina at Chapel Hill analyzed 30 years of scientific data to find out *why* Americans were eating 600 more calories per day in 2006 than they were in 1977. They discovered two main reasons: the increase in portion sizes; and the increase in the number of times per day we eat and drink.[8] During those 30 years, the average amount of food/drink consumed per "eating occasion" increased by 2.3 ounces per occasion. And those extra ounces add up pounds more quickly than ever, because we also had an average of 4.9 eating occasions per day in 2006, compared to 3.8 in 1977.

A few other alarming facts, courtesy of Brian Wansink, PhD, a professor at Cornell University and author of *Mindless Eating: Why We Eat More Than We Think*:[9]

- Jumbo-sized portions in restaurants, where we now spend more and more of every food dollar, are consistently 250% larger than regular portions. (And most items in fast-food restaurants are 2 to 5 times larger than they were 20 years ago, says the USDA.)
- People tend to eat 30% to 50% more from larger-sized restaurant portions, and 20% to 40% more from larger-sized packages. And eating a big portion today doesn't mean you'll turn one down tomorrow. In one study, normal and overweight people were served 50% larger portions over a period of 11 days and they overate day after day, for a grand total of 4,636 extra calories.
- The sizes of the glasses and bowls in our kitchens have steadily increased, and are now 36% larger than they were in 1960.

There are two main reasons why all of this supersizing causes us to overeat, according to Dr. Wansink:

- Larger packages, restaurant portions, and dinnerware have set a "consumption norm" that says it's "more appropriate, typical, reasonable, and normal" to eat larger portions.

- Large portions confuse us about how much we've actually eaten—you can eat a lot of food before you notice the amount has decreased! In one study, people ate 73% more tomato soup from bowls that were being secretly and imperceptibly refilled from underneath the table, compared to people eating from normal bowls—while estimating they ate only 5 calories more!

The Every-Other-Day Success Program helps you control portions by alternating the 1,000-calorie modified fast of Success Day with Feast Day—you don't overeat automatically. But to limit those portions can't hurt.

Science-based tips for portion control

Bill and I reviewed the last decade of studies on portion control to find the best, science-proven ways to help you manage portions on Success Day and Feast Day:

Use your plate to control your portions. Researchers at the Mayo Clinic studied 65 obese people, dividing them into two groups. For six months, one group used a "portion control plate" for their meals; they lost nearly five times more weight than those who did not use the plates.[10] In a similar six-month study, published in the *Archives of Internal Medicine*, obese people with type 2 diabetes using portion control plates lost 18 times more weight than a similar group not using the plates.[11]

In the Mayo study, the plate was clear glass with black print that divided it into three parts: one-half was labeled "vegetables"; one-quarter was labeled "fish, lean meat, chicken & nuts"; and one-quarter was labeled "potatoes, pasta, rice, beans and whole grains." The study participants were instructed to use the plate for their main meal and encouraged to use it for every meal.

I think dividing your meals into half vegetables and fruits, one-quarter protein, and one-quarter starch is a great (and easy) way to control your portions. Those portion sizes also match the latest recommendations from the USDA, where "MyPlate" (www.choosemyplate.gov) has replaced the food pyramid as the government's main nutritional advice. The USDA also recommends several daily servings of low-fat dairy; I think that's also a helpful strategy for weight maintenance.

You don't even have to *imagine* the portions: you can buy portion control plates like the kind used in the Mayo study, at every level of elegance and price, in retail stores and online. Examples include Lifestyle Dinner Plates from Precise Portions, the Portion Plate from beBetter Health, and Portion Conscious Dinner Plates from Slimware.

Increase the portion of fruits and vegetables. If you want to lower your calories, increase the portion of vegetables and fruits and decrease the portions of protein and starch. A study from researchers at Pennsylvania State University published in the *American Journal of Clinical Nutrition* showed that slightly increasing vegetables and slightly decreasing protein/starch decreased the overall calories of a meal by 14%.[12]

Serve food from smaller bowls. When people used a large bowl to serve pasta, they served 77% more than when using a medium-sized bowl, reported Dutch researchers in the *Journal of Nutrition Education and Behavior*.[13]

In a similar study, people given large bowls (34 ounces) and large ice-cream scoops (3 ounces) served themselves 53% more ice cream than people given medium-sized bowls (17 ounces) and medium scoops (2 ounces).

When people at a Super Bowl party were served from either a half-gallon or 1 gallon bowl, those eating from the larger bowl served themselves 53% more snacks—and ate 92% of what they'd served.

And when moviegoers were given free medium-sized or large buckets of popcorn to eat during the movie, those with the large buckets ate 51% more popcorn.

Buy smaller packages. "A shopper can buy smaller sizes, or create their own single-portion servings by subdividing the bargain-size bag into smaller ones," writes Dr. Wansink. During mealtime, keep the large packages or containers off the table and out of sight, he adds. That goes for beverages, too, of course. Research shows we get 21% of our daily calories from beverages, nearly *double* the amount in 1965.

Buy smaller snacks. People given 100-calorie snacks for a week ate 841 fewer calories from snacks compared to people given standard-size snacks, reported researchers from the University of Colorado.[14]

Order less at restaurants, or take some home. In one study, increasing a restaurant's portion size of pasta by one-third increased calorie intake by 43%, adding 172 more calories. "These results support the suggestion that large restaurant portions may be contributing to the obesity epidemic," wrote the researchers in *Obesity Research*.[15]

Don't count on well-meaning chefs to protect you. A study by researchers at Clemson University, published in *Obesity*, found that the majority of 300 executive chefs believed "large portions are a problem for weight control." Seventy-six percent of those chefs also claimed portions in their restaurants were "normal." But the researchers found that the portions of steak and pasta the chefs were actually serving were two to four times larger than the healthy portion sizes recommended by the government.[16]

What to do? "Consider splitting an entrée, or ordering an appetizer as your entrée, or having half the dinner packaged to go," advises Dr. Wansink.

Eat bigger portions of high-volume, low-calorie foods. Decreasing portion size by 25% led to a decreased mealtime intake of 231 calories in a meal, reported researchers from Pennsylvania State University. But so did *increasing* the portions of low-calorie, high-volume foods, like fruits, vegetables, soups, and low-fat milk—all of which allow you to eat and drink big portions of food *without* getting a lot of extra calories. "Reductions in both portion size and energy [calorie] density can help to moderate energy intake," wrote the researchers in the *American Journal of Clinical Nutrition*.[17]

Go to bed—you'll eat smaller portions tomorrow! Yes, getting enough Zzz's may mean eating smaller portions. In a study from Sweden, people who got less sleep chose breakfast portions that were 14% larger and midmorning snacks that were 16% larger, compared to people who had a good night's sleep.[18]

These changes and the diet and lifestyle tips in this chapter are for a *lifetime* of good health. No need to rush! If you make these changes slowly, you'll make them successfully. And you'll be rewarded by the intense satisfaction of being one of the few dieters who have lost weight and kept it off!

BARBARA'S STORY

Weight loss: 21 pounds

The campus of the University of Illinois-Chicago borders the Veterans Administration (VA) Medical Center, and a lot of VA nurses see the flyers advertising my studies and enroll in them; this included Barbara.

"People think nurses should know *everything* about health, but that's not how it is," she said with a smile. "I was sick, I was taking prednisone, I had gone up three dress sizes—and I just couldn't seem to make up my mind to stay on a diet. Then I saw the flyer for one of Dr. Varady's studies on alternate-day fasting and weight loss, and I decided that was for me."

After three months on the Every-Other-Day Diet, Barbara had lost 21 pounds. And she's kept it off—for 12 months.

"On Feast Day, I know I can eat anything—but I emphasize fruits and vegetables," she said. "My family knows I love fruit, and there's more fruit in the house than we ever had—melons, grapefruit, oranges, pomegranates, you name it."

She's also stopped eating fried foods, which she loved. "Now we cook a lot of food on the grill, even grilling vegetables and corn," she said.

And she started to walk. "I wear a pedometer and always take the stairs, and my office is on the fifth floor. And

(continued)

because the VA Medical Center is such a large place, I often walk between buildings, so it's not hard to get thousands of steps.

"I cheat sometimes on Success Day, but not often and never on two Success Days in a row," she said. "That's because my biggest fear is that I'll put the weight on again, so I do what I have to do to make sure that doesn't happen. I enjoy the compliments, and how good I feel, and my sense of accomplishment for having lost the weight and kept it off."

THE KEY WORD IN THE EOD SUCCESS PROGRAM IS *SUCCESS!*

Whether you bought this book to lose those last 5 or 10 pounds or an extra 20, 30, 40, or more; whether you've never dieted before or failed at every diet you've tried, I know you're going to find success with both the Every-Other-Day Diet and the Every-Other-Day Success Program. And I know it the way a scientist knows: because my careful, repeated studies show that the weight-loss and the weight-maintenance programs described in *The Every-Other-Day Diet* actually *work*.

The Every-Other-Day Diet works to help you lose weight—whatever your weight-loss goal, I know you'll reach it!

The Every-Other-Day Success Program works to help you keep the weight off—if you follow the program, I know you won't regain the pounds you shed.

It's been my pleasure to bring the EOD Diet and Success

Program from the pages of scientific journals to the pages of this book, and into your life. Bill and I wish you the best, for a trim and healthy life!

EOD—Easy as 1-2-3!

1. On the EOD Success Program, you eat 1,000 calories on Monday, Wednesday, and Friday, and you eat whatever you want the other days of the week.
2. Mindful eating—slowing down and paying attention to your meal, bite by bite—is a proven key to weight maintenance.
3. Portion control—at home and wherever else you eat—is one of the best ways to control calories.

Acknowledgments

From Dr. Krista Varady:

I would like to thank my coauthor, Bill Gottlieb; literary agent, Chris Tomasino; and editor, Christine Pride, for all of their hard work, support, and encouragement throughout this process. I am also grateful to Peter Jones and Marc Hellerstein for their outstanding mentorship during my doctoral and postdoctoral degrees. Last, I would like to thank my doctoral students—Surabhi Bhutani, Monica Klempel, Cynthia Kroeger, John Trepanowski, and Kristin Hoddy—for their diligent work in coordinating all of the human trials discussed in this book.

From Bill Gottlieb:

A finished book is an occasion for expressing a lot of gratitude, because so many people (too many to thank here!) have contributed to its creation and completion. But special thanks must go to...

My co-author, Dr. Krista Varady, for her groundbreaking research, lively intelligence, and constant collegiality: Krista, you were the perfect collaborator! To Stephanie Karpinske, for her excellent (and fast!) work in producing the recipes for the book, and for providing an abundance of advice about frozen foods. To Christine Tomasino, my literary agent of 15 years, who has brought her creativity, energy, canny nego-tiating, and consistent care to each of the 15 books I've writ-ten: Chris, I can't thank you enough. To our literary lawyer, Heather Florence, for all her careful, crucial, protective work on behalf of this project. To Matt Inman, our acquisition edi-tor at Hyperion Books; and to Liz Gough, our acquisition editor at Hodder. To Christine Pride, our superb editor, who worked at super-speed, with super-skill, and improved the book immeasurably. To Gretchen Young at Hachette, for all her diligence and kindness; thank you for making sure the manuscript kept moving! And a final thank you to all the other members of the editorial team at Hachette who brought their unique skills to producing this book.

Notes

Chapter 1

1. Gardner, C. D., et al. "Comparison of the Atkins, Zone, Ornish, and LEARN Diets for Change in Weight and Related Risk Factors among Overweight Premenopausal Women: The A TO Z Weight Loss Study: A Randomized Trial." *Journal of the American Medical Association* 297, no. 9 (March 7, 2007): 969–77.

2. Heilbronn, L. K., et al. "Alternate-Day Fasting in Nonobese Subjects: Effects on Body Weight, Body Composition, and Energy Metabolism." *American Journal of Clinical Nutrition* 81, no. 1 (January 2005): 69–73.

3. Varady, K. A., et al. "Short-Term Modified Alternate-Day Fasting: A Novel Dietary Strategy for Weight Loss and Cardioprotection in Obese Adults." *American Journal of Clinical Nutrition* 90 (2009): 1138–43.

4. Ibid.

5. Klempel, M. C., et al. "Dietary and Physical Activity Adaptations to Alternate Day Modified Fasting: Implications for Optimal Weight Loss." *Nutrition Journal* 9 (2010): 35.

6. Bhutani, S., et al. "Improvements in Coronary Heart Disease Risk Indicators by Alternate-Day Fasting Involve Adipose Tissue Modulations." *Obesity* 18, no. 11 (November 2010): 2152–59.

7. Klempel, M. C., et al. "Alternate Day Fasting (ADF) with a High-Fat Diet Produces Similar Weight Loss and Cardio-Protection as

ADF with a Low-Fat Diet." *Metabolism* 62, no. 1 (January 2013): 137–43.

8. Bhutani, S., et al. "Alternate Day Fasting and Endurance Exercise Combine to Reduce Body Weight and Favorably Alter Plasma Lipids on Obese Humans." *Obesity* (February 14, 2013).

9. Kramer, F. M., et al. "Long-Term Follow-Up of Behavioral Treatment for Obesity: Patterns of Weight Regain among Men and Women." *International Journal of Obesity* 13, no. 2 (1989): 123–36.

Chapter 2

1. VanWormer, J. J., et al. "Self-Weighing Promotes Weight Loss for Obese Adults." *American Journal of Preventive Medicine* 36, no. 1 (January 2009): 70–73.

2. VanWormer, J. J., et al. "Self-Weighing Frequency Is Associated with Weight Gain Prevention over 2 Years among Working Adults." *International Journal of Behavioral Medicine* 19, no. 3 (September 2012): 351–58.

3. Steinberg, D. M., et al. "The Efficacy of a Daily Self-Weighing Weight Loss Intervention Using Smart Scales and Email." *Obesity* (March 20, 2013).

4. Butryn, M. L., et al. "Consistent Self-Monitoring of Weight: A Key Component of Successful Weight Loss Maintenance." *Obesity* 15, no. 12 (December 2007): 3091–96.

5. Linde, J. A., et al. "Self-Weighing in Weight Gain Prevention and Weight Loss Trials." *Annals of Behavioral Medicine* 30, no. 3 (December 2005): 210–16.

6. Douglas, S. M., et al. "Low, Moderate, or High Protein Yogurt Snacks on Appetite Control and Subsequent Eating in Healthy Women." *Appetite* 60, no. 1 (January 2013): 117–22.

7. Leidy, H. J., et al. "The Influence of Higher Protein Intake and Greater Eating Frequency on Appetite Control in Overweight and Obese Men." *Obesity* 18, no. 9 (September 2010): 1725–32.

8. Mozaffarian, D., et al. "Plasma Phospholipid Long-Chain ω-3 Fatty Acids and Total and Cause-Specific Mortality in Older Adults: A Cohort Study." *Annals of Internal Medicine* 158, no. 7 (April 2013): 515–25.

9. Estruch, R., et al. "Primary Prevention of Cardiovascular Disease with a Mediterranean Diet." *New England Journal of Medicine* 368, no. 14 (April 2013): 1279–90.

10. Siri-Tarino, P. W., et al. "Meta-Analysis of Prospective Cohort Studies Evaluating the Association of Saturated Fat with Cardiovascular Disease." *American Journal of Clinical Nutrition* 91, no. 3 (March 2010): 535–46.

11. Kong, A., et al. "Associations between Snacking and Weight Loss and Nutrient Intake among Postmenopausal Overweight to Obese Women in a Dietary Weight-Loss Intervention." *Journal of the American Dietetic Association* 111, no. 12 (December 2011): 1898–903.

12. Hibi, M., et al. "Nighttime Snacking Reduces Whole Body Fat Oxidation and Increases LDL Cholesterol in Healthy Young Women." *American Journal of Physiology: Regulatory, Integrative and Comparative Physiology* 304, no. 2 (January 2013): R94–R101.

13. Stroebele, N., et al. "Do Calorie-Controlled Portion Sizes of Snacks Reduce Energy Intake?" *Appetite* 52, no. 3 (June 2009): 793–96.

14. Zizza, C. A., and B. Xu. "Snacking Is Associated with Overall Diet Quality among Adults." *Journal of the Academy of Nutrition and Dietetics* 112, no. 2 (February 2012): 291–96.

15. Zizza, C. A., et al. "Contribution of Snacking to Older Adults' Vitamin, Carotenoid, and Mineral Intakes." *Journal of the American Dietetic Association* 110, no. 5 (May 2010): 768–72.

16. Bachman, J. L., et al. "Eating Frequency Is Higher in Weight Loss Maintainers and Normal-Weight Individuals Than in Overweight Individuals." *Journal of the American Dietetic Association* 111, no. 11 (November 2011): 1730–34.

17. Van Walleghen, E. L., et al. "Pre-Meal Water Consumption Reduces Meal Energy Intake in Older but Not Younger Subjects." *Obesity* 15, no. 1 (January 2007): 93–99.

18. Davy, B. M., et al. "Water Consumption Reduces Energy Intake at a Breakfast Meal in Obese Older Adults." *Journal of the American Dietetic Association* 108, no. 7 (July 2008): 1236–39.

19. Boschmann, M., et al. "Water Drinking Induces Thermogenesis through Osmosensitive Mechanisms." *Journal of Clinical Endocrinology and Metabolism* 92, no. 8 (August 2007): 3334–37.

20. Akers, J. D., et al. "Daily Self-Monitoring of Body Weight, Step Count, Fruit/Vegetable Intake, and Water Consumption: A Feasible and Effective Long-Term Weight Loss Maintenance Approach." *Journal of the Academy of Nutrition and Dietetics* 112, no. 5 (May 2012): 685–692.

21. Rudenga, K. J., et al. "Amygdala Response to Sucrose Consumption Is Inversely Related to Artificial Sweetener Use." *Appetite* 58, no. 2 (April 2012): 504–7.

22. Fowler, S. P., et al. "Fueling the Obesity Epidemic? Artificially Sweetened Beverage Use and Long-Term Weight Gain." *Obesity* 16, no. 8 (August 2008): 1894–900.

23. Bernstein, A. M., et al. "Soda Consumption and the Risk of Stroke in Men and Women." *American Journal of Clinical Nutrition* 95, no. 5 (May 2012): 1190–99.

24. Schernhammer, E. S., et al. "Consumption of Artificial Sweetener- and Sugar-Containing Soda and Risk of Lymphoma and Leukemia in Men and Women." *American Journal of Clinical Nutrition* 96, no. 6 (December 2012): 1419–28.

25. Nettleton, J. A., et al. "Diet Soda Intake and Risk of Incident Metabolic Syndrome and Type 2 Diabetes in the Multi-Ethnic Study of Atherosclerosis (MESA)." *Diabetes Care* 32, no. 4 (April 2009): 688–94.

26. Karalius, V. P., et al. "Dietary Sugar and Artificial Sweetener Intake and Chronic Kidney Disease: A Review." *Advances in Chronic Kidney Disease* 20, no. 2 (March 2013): 157–64.

27. Pepino, M. Y., et al. "Sucralose Affects Glycemic and Hormonal Responses to an Oral Glucose Load." *Diabetes Care* (April 30, 2013).

28. Gavrieli, A., et al. "Effect of Different Amounts of Coffee on Dietary Intake and Appetite of Normal-Weight and Overweight/Obese Individuals." *Obesity* (November 29, 2012).

29. Lopez-Garcia, E., et al. "Changes in Caffeine Intake and Long-Term Weight Change in Men and Women." *American Journal of Clinical Nutrition* 83, no. 3 (March 2006): 674–80.

30. Carter, B. E., et al. "Beverages Containing Soluble Fiber, Caffeine, and Green Tea Catechins Suppress Hunger and Lead to Less Energy Consumption at the Next Meal." *Appetite* 59, no. 3 (December 2012): 755–61.

31. Hursel, R., et al. "The Effects of Green Tea on Weight Loss and Weight Maintenance: A Meta-Analysis." *International Journal of Obesity* 33, no. 9 (September 2009): 956–61.

32. Freedman, N. D., et al. "Association of Coffee Drinking with Total and Cause-Specific Mortality." *New England Journal of Medicine* 366, no. 20 (May 2012): 1891–904.

33. Hetherington, M. M., et al. "Effects of Chewing Gum on Short-Term Appetite Regulation in Moderately Restrained Eaters." *Appetite* 57, no. 2 (October 2011): 475–82.

34. Smith, A. P., et al. "Effects of Chewing Gum on the Stress and Work of University Students." *Appetite* 58, no. 3 (June 2012): 1037–40.

35. Zibell, S., et al. "Impact of Gum Chewing on Stress Levels: Online Self-Perception Research Study." *Current Medical Research and Opinion* 25, no. 6 (June 2009): 1491–500.

36. Scholey, A., et al. "Chewing Gum Alleviates Negative Mood and Reduces Cortisol during Acute Laboratory Psychological Stress." *Physiology & Behavior* 97, no. 3–4 (June 2009): 304–12.

Chapter 4

1. Unlu, N. Z., et al. "Carotenoid Absorption from Salad and Salsa by Humans Is Enhanced by the Addition of Avocado or Avocado Oil." *Journal of Nutrition* 135, no. 3 (March 2005): 431–36.

2. Johnston, C. S., et al. "Vinegar: Medicinal Uses and Antiglycemic Effect." *Mescape General Medicine* 8, no. 2 (May 30, 2006): 61.

3. Tedong, L., et al. "Hydro-Ethanolic Extract of Cashew Tree (Anacardium Occidentale) Nut and Its Principal Compound, Anacardic Acid, Stimulate Glucose Uptake in C2C12 Muscle Cells." *Molecular Nutrition and Food Research* 54, no. 12 (December 2010): 1753–62.

4. Kamil, A., et al. "Health Benefits of Almonds beyond Cholesterol Reduction." *Journal of Agricultural and Food Chemistry* (February 17, 2012).

5. Russo, M., et al. "The Flavonoid Quercetin in Disease Prevention and Therapy." *Biochemical Pharmacology* 83, no. 1 (January 1, 2012): 6–15.

6. Mellen, P. B., et al. "Whole Grain Intake and Cardiovascular Disease: A Meta-Analysis." *Nutrition, Metabolism and Cardiovascular Diseases* 18, no. 4 (May 2008): 283–90.

7. Reis, C. E., et al. "Ground Roasted Peanuts Leads to a Lower Post-Prandial Glycemic Response Than Raw Peanuts." *Nutrition Hospital* 26, no. 4 (July–August 2011): 745–51.

8. Oude Griep, L. M., et al. "Colors of Fruit and Vegetables and 10-Year Incidence of Stroke." *Stroke* 42, no. 11 (November 2011): 3190–95.

9. Shardell, M. D., et al. "Low-Serum Carotenoid Concentrations and Carotenoid Interactions Predict Mortality in US Adults: The Third National Health and Nutrition Examination Survey." *Nutrition Research* 31, no. 3 (March 2011): 178–89.

10. Butt, M. S., et al. "Black Pepper and Health Claims: A Comprehensive Treatise." *Critical Reviews in Food Science and Nutrition* 53, no. 9 (2013): 875–86.

11. Russell, F. D., et al. "Distinguishing Health Benefits of Eicosapentaenoic and Docosahexaenoic Acids." *Marine Drugs* 10, no. 11 (November 13, 2012): 2535–59.

12. Ludy, M. J., et al. "The Effects of Capsaicin and Capsiate on Energy Balance: Critical Review and Meta-Analyses of Studies in Humans." *Chemical Senses* 37, no. 2 (February 2012): 103–21.

13. Ratliff, J., et al. "Consuming Eggs for Breakfast Influences Plasma Glucose and Ghrelin, while Reducing Energy Intake during the Next 24 Hours in Adult Men." *Nutrition Research* 30, no. 2 (February 2010): 96–103.

14. Xu, Y., et al. "Effect of Dietary Supplementation with White Button Mushrooms on Host Resistance to Influenza Infection and Immune Function in Mice." *British Journal of Nutrition* 109, no. 6 (March 28, 2013): 1052–61.

15. Diliberti, N., et al. "Increased Portion Size Leads to Increased Energy Intake in a Restaurant Meal." *Obesity* 12, no. 3 (March 2004): 562–68.

16. Hettiaratchi, U. P., et al. "Chemical Compositions and Glycemic Responses to Banana Varieties." *International Journal of Food Sciences and Nutrition* 62, no. 4 (June 2011): 307–9.

17. Katz, D. L., et al. "Cocoa and Chocolate in Human Health and Disease." *Antioxidants and Redox Signaling* 15, no. 10 (November 2011): 2779–811.

18. Patel, B. P., et al. "An After-School Snack of Raisins Lowers Cumulative Food Intake in Young Children." *Journal of Food Science* 78, no. S1 (June 2013): A5–A10.

19. Akilen, R., et al. "Cinnamon in Glycaemic Control: Systematic Review and Meta Analysis." *Clinical Nutrition* 31, no. 5 (October 2012): 609–15.

20. Cesar, T. B., et al. "Orange Juice Decreases Low-Density Lipoprotein Cholesterol in Hypercholesterolemic Subjects and Improves Lipid Transfer to High-Density Lipoprotein in Normal and Hypercholesterolemic Subjects." *Nutrition Research* 30, no. 10 (October 2010): 689–94.

21. Kurowska, E. M., et al. "HDL-Cholesterol-Raising Effect of Orange Juice in Subjects with Hypercholesterolemia." *American Journal of Clinical Nutrition* 72, no. 5 (November 2000): 1095–100.

22. Zhang, Y., et al. "Cherry Consumption and Decreased Risk of Recurrent Gout Attacks." *Arthritis and Rheumatism* 64, no. 12 (December 2012): 4004–11.

23. Kelley, D. S., et al. "Sweet Bing Cherries Lower Circulating Concentrations of Markers for Chronic Inflammatory Diseases in Healthy Humans." *Journal of Nutrition* 143, no. 3 (March 2013): 340–44.

24. Howatson, G., et al. "Effect of Tart Cherry Juice (Prunus Cerasus) on Melatonin Levels and Enhanced Sleep Quality." *European Journal of Nutrition* 51, no. 8 (December 2012): 909–16.

25. Moazzami, A. A., et al. "Metabolomics Reveals the Metabolic Shifts Following an Intervention with Rye Bread in Postmenopausal Women—A Randomized Control Trial." *Nutrition Journal* 11 (October 2012): 88.

26. Basu, A., et al. "Strawberries Decrease Atherosclerotic Markers in Subjects with Metabolic Syndrome." *Nutrition Research* 30, no. 7 (July 2010): 462–69.

27. Nguyen, V., et al. "Popcorn Is More Satiating Than Potato Chips in Normal-Weight Adults." *Nutrition Journal* 11 (September 14, 2012): 71.

Chapter 6

1. Bhutani, S., et al. "Alternate Day Fasting and Endurance Exercise Combine to Reduce Body Weight and Favorably Alter Plasma Lipids on Obese Humans." *Obesity* (February 14, 2013).
2. Bassett, D. R., Jr., et al. "Pedometer-Measured Physical Activity and Health Behaviors in U.S. Adults." *Medicine and Science in Sports and Exercise* 42, no. 10 (October 2010): 1819–25.
3. Hultquist, C. N., et al. "Comparison of Walking Recommendations in Previously Inactive Women." *Medicine and Science in Sports and Exercise* 37, no. 4 (April 2005): 676–83.
4. Tudor-Locke, C., et al. "The Relationship between Pedometer-Determined Ambulatory Activity and Body Composition Variables." *International Journal of Obesity and Related Metabolic Disorders* 25, no. 11 (November 2001): 1571–78.
5. Bravata, D. M., "Using Pedometers to Increase Physical Activity and Improve Health: A Systematic Review." *Journal of the American Medical Association* 298, no. 19 (November 21, 2007): 2296–304.
6. Croteau, K. A. "Strategies Used to Increase Lifestyle Physical Activity in a Pedometer-Based Intervention." *Journal of Allied Health* 33, no. 4 (Winter 2004): 278–81.
7. Steeves, J. A., et al. "Can Sedentary Behavior Be Made More Active? A Randomized Pilot Study of TV Commercial Stepping Versus Walking." *International Journal of Behavioral Nutrition and Physical Activity* 9 (August 6, 2012): 95.

Chapter 7

1. "ObesityWeek 2013," a presentation at the yearly scientific conference of the American Society for Metabolic and Bariatric Surgery, which publishes the journal *Obesity*, of first-year results from a three-year study sponsored by the National Institutes of Health.

2. Mekary, R. A., et al. "Physical Activity in Relation to Long-Term Weight Maintenance After Intentional Weight Loss in Premenopausal Women. *Obesity* 18, no. 1 (January 2010): 167–74.

3. Robinson, E., et al. "Eating Attentively: A Systematic Review and Meta-Analysis of the Effect of Food Intake Memory and Awareness on Eating." *American Journal of Clinical Nutrition* 97, no. 4 (April 2013): 728–42.

4. Beshara, M., et al. "Does Mindfulness Matter? Everyday Mindfulness, Mindful Eating and Self-Reported Serving Size of Energy Dense Foods among a Sample of South Australian Adults." *Appetite* 67 (August 2013): 25–29.

5. Alberts, H. J., et al. "Dealing with Problematic Eating Behaviour: The Effects of a Mindfulness-Based Intervention on Eating Behaviour, Food Cravings, Dichotomous Thinking and Body Image Concern." *Appetite* 58, no. 3 (June 2012): 847–51.

6. Paolini, B., et al. "Coping with Brief Periods of Food Restriction: Mindfulness Matters." *Frontiers in Aging Neuroscience* 4 (2012): 13.

7. Daubenmier, J., et al. "Mindfulness Intervention for Stress Eating to Reduce Cortisol and Abdominal Fat among Overweight and Obese Women: An Exploratory Randomized Controlled Study." *Journal of Obesity* (2011): Article ID 651936.

8. Duffey, K. J., et al. "Energy Density, Portion Size, and Eating Occasions: Contributions to Increased Energy Intake in the United States, 1977–2006." *PLoS Medicine* 8, no. 6 (June 2011): e1001050.

9. Wansink, B., et al. "Portion Size Me: Downsizing Our Consumption Norms." *Journal of the American Dietetic Association, Journal of the American Dietetic Association* 107, no. 7 (July 2007): 1103–6.

10. Kesman, R. L., et al. "Portion Control for the Treatment of Obesity in the Primary Care Setting." *BMC Research Notes* 4 (September 9, 2011): 346.

11. Pedersen, S. D., et al. "Portion Control Plate for Weight Loss in Obese Patients with Type 2 Diabetes Mellitus: A Controlled

Clinical Trial." *Archives of Internal Medicine* 167, no. 12 (June 2007): 1277–83.

12. Rolls, B. J., et al. "Portion Size Can Be Used Strategically to Increase Vegetable Consumption in Adults." *American Journal of Clinical Nutrition* 91, no. 4 (April 2010): 913–22.

13. Van Kleef, E., et al. "Serving Bowl Selection Biases the Amount of Food Served." *Journal of Nutrition Education and Behavior* 44, no. 1 (January–February 2012): 66–70.

14. Stroebele, N., et al. "Do Calorie-Controlled Portion Sizes of Snacks Reduce Energy Intake?" *Appetite* 52, no. 3 (June 2009): 793–96.

15. Rolls, B. J., et al. "Salad and Satiety: Energy Density and Portion Size of a First-Course Salad Affect Energy Intake at Lunch." *Journal of the American Dietetic Association* 104, no. 10 (October 2004): 1570–76.

16. Condrasky, M., et al. "Chefs' Opinions of Restaurant Portion Sizes." *Obesity* 15, no. 8 (August 2007): 2086–94.

17. Rolls, B. J., et al. "Portion Size Can Be Used Strategically to Increase Vegetable Consumption in Adults." *American Journal of Clinical Nutrition* 91, no. 4 (April 2010): 913–22.

18. Hogenkamp, P. S., et al. "Acute Sleep Deprivation Increases Portion Size and Affects Food Choice in Young Men." *Psychoneuroendocrinology* 38, no. 9 (September 2013): 1668–74.

Index